HEALTHY
BY CHOICE
Your Blueprint for Vital Living

Shawna Curry RN, BN, BKin

PRAISE FOR *HEALTHY BY CHOICE*

"As a Primary Care Physician, I take care of patients of all ages who suffer from all types of acute and chronic illnesses. More and more, I have been seeing patients whose chronic disease and symptoms are the result of years of stress and poor lifestyle choices. It is time we stopped practicing "sick care" and moved to teaching patients the fundamentals of Wellness. Shawna's new book provides patients the prescription they need to stop struggling with fad diets and take charge of their own health. It's not about short-term diets that don't work, it's about a whole LIFESTYLE change. I can only hope that all of my patients read this book and start enacting these changes in their life. It will be available in my office for everyone!"

—Pamela A McGrogan, MD, Board Certified Family Medicine,
Obesity and Lifestyle Medicine Practitioner

"There is so much information available and recommendations constantly bombarding us. Shawna has done the reading for us and talent the best evidence based, scientific recommendations and explained them in an achievable way. She has paved a path to safe and healthy life choices."

— Heidi Osborne, Physiotherapist, Evidence Sport and Spine

"Healthy by Choice should be required reading for anyone who wants to stay active, mobile and energized to the end of their days. Without addressing the 7 Pillars of Health, so clearly laid out in this book, the body may not be ready for the activity required to maintain the high quality of life we envision for ourselves. This book provides not only the pillars, but the foundation to build a happy home within bodies."

—Wendy Coombs BSc.PT, BSc.Psych; Physiotherapist,
CEO Momentum Health/Evidence Sport & Spine/
Innovative Sport Medicine

"Shawna has written an informative, fun, engaging, insightful, and thought-provoking book covering a broad range of health and wellness topics. This will be a great resource for someone looking to get a grip on all aspects of their health. I would not hesitate to recommend this book to my patients, colleagues, other health professionals."

—Ian Goodwin, BScPT, FCAMPT, cGIMS, MATS, Co-Owner,
Physiotherapist, Calgary Core Physiotherapy

"Shawna's practical, realistic and manageable approach has helped me design wellness on my terms. After years of inconsistent weight loss and gain, I finally feel like I can trust the innate knowing of my body to steer me in the right direction."

—Karen Rowe, #1 International Bestselling Author,
Owner, Front Rowe Seat

"Shawna is a no-B.S. woman. What I love about this book is she avoided giving us the 'quick fix' and instead, went with the 'real fix.' It speaks directly to the heart of why women often fail to achieve the success and freedom they want. I am so grateful I now have a resource I can give to any of my friends or family who are tired of the same old advice and want the truth about chronic disease and weight gain."

—Jordan Reasoner, Co-Founder, SCD Lifestyle

Editorial Project Management: Karen Rowe, Karen@KarenRowe.com

Cover Design: Shake Creative, ShakeTampa.com

Inside Layout: Ljiljana Pavkov

Printed in the United States

ISBN: 978-1-7750744-0-3 (international trade paper edition)

ISBN: 978-1-7750744-1-0 (ebook)

Published by The Lifestyle Strategy

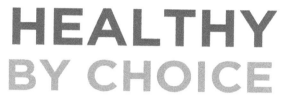

HEALTHY
BY CHOICE
Your Blueprint for Vital Living

Table of Contents

As a special bonus for purchasing this book, you are invited to join a private Facebook group specifically designed to enhance your experience. I know that you'll get better results if you have a support network. The Facebook community is there for you to connect with like-minded individuals that will help you stay accountable for your goals and to inspire you to take action. I'll personally pop on the group site to offer tips and feedback to help guide you to greater success.

To gain access to this private community, go to

www.facebook.com/groups/blueprintforvitalliving

See you inside!

Foreword

*T*he first thing you will notice as you start reading this extremely valuable book is the authenticity of the author, Shawna Curry. I like that.

You can find numerous "quick-fix" health and diet books on the market these days that make wild promises and offer instant remedies for all sorts of ailments; it's overwhelming!

Shawna obviously has a genuine passion for helping people. She even changed careers to ensure that her future would be dedicated to serving others in the most meaningful way. Her commitment to uncovering the truth about healthy living shines throughout the entire book.

This is no quick makeover that only touches the surface of serious health issues. The author digs deep, delving into sound research and practical remedies that can transform your life.

I also appreciate the fact that there are lots of Action Steps and questions that make you stop and think. You will quickly become engaged in examining your current lifestyle to determine what's working and what needs to be improved. Shawna guides you through this process in a friendly, encouraging manner.

What reinforces everything is the story of Shawna's own significant health and mental challenges and her long battle to find the right solutions. No fluffy concepts or theory here; this is real life portrayed in a way that will inspire you and create a high level of trust and confidence.

I've had the good fortune to be mentored by some outstanding mentors and teachers in my journey through life. None of those people "dabbled" at improving themselves and others. They were "all in" and proved to be great role models who always led by example. Shawna has that same level of determination to add real value to the audience she serves.

You'll find this book easy to read, too. There are plenty of excellent analogies and stories to deepen your understanding. By distilling your overall health into seven distinct areas, you can select what's most important to you and start working on it right away. The section on sleep alone is worth the price of the book!

As Shawna reminds us, we are ultimately responsible for the choices we make. I encourage you to choose wisely from this treasury of "health wealth" and reap the rewards. Failing to do so can create circumstances that will be totally out of your control. And "health poverty" is no fun at all!

Les Hewitt
#1 New York Times bestselling author, *The Power of Focus*
Founder of the kidsED project
leshewitt.com

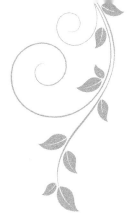

Preface

Back in 1988, the Surgeon General's Report on Nutrition and Health indicated that the most common diseases in the United States were high blood pressure, coronary artery disease, cancers, diabetes, and obesity. In 2003, the World Health Organization (WHO) confirmed the same.

Today, we have more dietary and lifestyle recommendations than ever before, yet nothing has changed. Instead, the rates of these chronic diseases are rising in number every year. All those dietary and lifestyle recommendations clearly aren't working!

What's alarming is that all of these diseases are *preventable* conditions linked to unhealthy lifestyle habits. The WHO cites that the cost of chronic diseases accounts for approximately 46 percent of the global burden of disease, with that number anticipated to increase to 57 percent by 2020. To help ease this burden, they suggest, "primary prevention is considered to be the most cost-effective, affordable, and sustainable course of action to cope with the chronic disease epidemic worldwide."

What is primary prevention? Essentially, it's preventing disease *before* it starts. Instead of trying to "catch it early" and lessen the impact of a condition, primary prevention is about engaging in activities that are well researched and proven to *prevent* diseases from occurring in the first place. That's the focus of this book. To focus on improving your health now rather than reacting to a diagnosis later.

By investing in primary prevention, you'll be able to get a significant return on your investment. Studies show that for every dollar you invest in prevention, you'll get between three to five dollars back in cost savings down the road.

Why, then, isn't there a rush of people signing up to be proactive? The WHO suggests this is due to a number of factors, including "underestimation of the effectiveness of interventions, the belief of there being a long delay in achieving any measurable impact, commercial pressures, institutional inertia, and inadequate resources."

Rather than waiting for more research studies to come out telling you other reasons to adopt a healthy lifestyle, start today.

With over sixteen years of experience working as a nurse, personal trainer, and coach and leading presentations on various health and nutrition topics, I have noticed a trend in the types of questions that are asked over and over again. Information that seems like common sense to me, I have realized, is not so common.

In a world where obesity has become an epidemic and chronic disease rates are soaring, I switched careers to become a nurse in order to gain credibility and affect greater change. As my passion for promoting health and fitness has grown, I have sought out more effective ways of sharing this information, and writing a book seemed the best way to touch as many people as possible.

As a nurse, I'm taught to use information that is *research-based* or to use *evidence-based medicine* when teaching my patients. This is part of my ethical code that I agree to each year when I renew my nursing license. I was also encouraged to use this same *quality* information as a kinesiologist and personal trainer, though not bound by the same level of ethics. Unfortunately, what I have found over my years of practice and through my use of such *evidence-based research* is that the information presented is not always up to date on the newest research and is not always in the best interest of the patient.

My health recommendations relate to seven key pillars: Sleep, Nutrition, Exercise, Mental Health, Digestion, Medical Conditions, and Lifestyle Factors. In order to be optimally healthy, you *need* these areas to be in balance. I didn't just make them up; they keep coming up in the literature—over and over again!

I've spent years going through hundreds of journal articles discovering low and high recommendations for each of these areas, and have summarized the facts for you. I evaluated guidelines put together by governments (Canada's Food Guide, USDA My Plate), health organizations (Canadian Diabetes Association, Heart and Stroke Foundation), functional medicine, ancestral living, natural nutrition, evolutionary psychology, you name it! These recommendations are designed for individuals like you who aren't just satisfied with a *so-so* quality of life. You want and deserve better.

You want to achieve optimal health. This book is not a new fad diet or lifestyle, but rather, a way of looking at your current lifestyle and adjusting it to optimize your health. It includes adding foods that give your body more nutrients to heal itself and removing foods that are creating inflammation.

Similar to cooking, you have to follow the recipe to achieve success. I'm one of those cooks who takes their own liberties and changes the ingredients because I think other spices or varied measurements will result in a better recipe. By the time I'm done cooking, the recipe is completely different. Changing lifestyle habits follows the same idea. Many people will go on diets or exercise programs and end up *cheating* or making up their own rules, and then complain that they didn't get results. They become defensive and resistant to making future changes.

In the health industry, quick fixes are commonplace, but you won't find those here. What you will find in this book is information to provide you with a general understanding of health topics including nutrition, sleep, mental health, and exercise. My goal is to challenge your current way of thinking about your health, and to define ways for you to make simple changes that will provide you with greater health, improved fitness, increased energy, and lasting vitality. Specifically, you will learn how to make healthier food choices, increase your activity level, and employ stress reduction techniques to enjoy a well-balanced lifestyle without feeling deprived like you do on most programs. You will learn how to plan your own strategy to lose weight, change your body composition, and improve your health in a way that is achievable and long-lasting.

As with any time you make changes to your lifestyle, you may experience setbacks or failures. You can use those experiences to find your own inner strength and continue your progress rather than falling back into old habits. There are several activities to do throughout this book that will guide your progress and keep you on track. I encourage you to spend time on each of them to focus on your personal goals so that you may truly make lasting changes.

Over the years, many of my clients and patients have said that they wished someone had told them that they needed to change their lifestyle and that unhealthy habits were putting their health/lives at risk. So here's my wake-up call for you. You need to change! You are bombarded by messages telling you it's not your fault—it's just your genetics, the environment, or your metabolism. Truthfully, all of those factors matter, as well as everything you do day in and day out that has an influence on how healthy you are.

Here's your chance to take charge of your life and make lasting changes to be healthier, stronger, leaner, and more energetic. If you aren't ready to make some changes—don't go any further. Please come back and read this book when you *are* truly ready to change your life. You'll need to be ready to put in the effort in order to obtain lasting changes. Your bad habits won't change themselves! If you are reading this book in hopes of trying to make someone else change—good luck, it won't happen. You can present the book as a gift, but understand that they will only initiate change when they are truly ready.

This is a book that has changed my life. The things I have learned about myself while on my journey to health are beyond what I thought possible. Not only have I learned a lot more than I thought I already knew about health, nutrition, and exercise, but I have learned so much more about myself. I have learned to love my body with all its perfect imperfections,

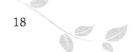

and have become more confident and comfortable in my own skin. I've learned to feel attractive, beautiful, and sexy, because I am. Now, I truly love myself and my body for what it is. Mine. Because I deserve it all. I am worth all of it.

This is a book that has changed my life. I hope it will change yours too. I wish you good luck on your journey to better health!

Acknowledgements

This book would never have happened if it weren't for Jason-the-dream-crusher. When I thought my loving husband, Jason was being critical and crushing my dream of writing a book, he was actually being supportive. It took us a while to see eye-to-eye and get on the same page, but eventually, "Jason-the-dream-crusher" became a pet name for my husband when he wanted to offer constructive feedback. Jason challenged me to consider *why* my book would be different than every other book out there, which allowed me to work through the process on a deeper level and write a much better book. Thank you to both my husband Jason and Jason-the-dream-crusher!

For giving me the initial confidence and believing in my ability to write a book back when I was in high school, I thank my English teacher Mrs. Jordan. The initial inspiration for this book came from Les Hewitt, author of *The Power of Focus*, who made a profound impact on my life without even knowing it. Your words will stick with me forever. Thank you to my coach Heather Wilde for your encouragement and ability to help me realize my dreams. Your guidance and support helped me push through when I was ready to give up.

Thank you to my family and friends, who listened to me *talk* about writing a book for ten years before I started to actually *write* a book—thank you for your support over the many, many years. Thank you to my colleagues who offered their thoughts, insights, expertise, and direction to resources to add more value to each topic discussed in this book. Each of you has influenced my book in many ways.

A special thank you to my editors Karen Rowe and Corey McCullough for your support and feedback, which helped to pull my rambling, incoherent thoughts together into a much better product. Your patience with my procrastination as I kept making major changes in the development phase was much appreciated. Thank you for helping me to realize that I was able to write a book in a much shorter timeline than I ever thought possible.

My final thank you goes out to the many individuals who have helped to influence my work: Jason Ahlan, Marissa Atkinson, Wendy Coombs, Giulia Enders, Kate Fitzpatrick, Sarah Fragoso, Pilar Gerasimo, Ian Goodwin, Dallas Hartwig, Lisa Hildebrand, Maryjane Kapteyn, Chris Kresser, Eric Lavoie, Megan McElheran, Tammy Moroz, Bryan Myles, Heidi Osborne, Joe Polish, Michael Pollan, Jennifer Powter, Marie Rayma, Jordan Reasoner, Diane Sanfilippo, Masoud Shahanaghi, Robin Sharma, Gary Taubes, Barb Thomas, Greg Uchacz, Jay Winans, Robb Wolf, Frankie Wong, and Steve Wright.

Introduction

I'd like to share with you a bit of my background to help you understand where some of my passion for health and fitness comes from. I grew up as a very skinny kid, with people always telling me that I needed to "put some meat on my bones." I never really had any major health issues growing up, other than getting chicken pox two times, but I did struggle from temper tantrums as a child and mood swings as a teenager. I never really attributed my moods to anything in particular, nor did my parents.

Despite being generally healthy, I had a significant overbite that was identified when I was only three years old, which was followed by regular visits to an orthodontist from then onwards. Growing up, I suffered from TMJ pain along with the clicking and locking of my jaw that got so bad that I needed surgical correction to enable me to continue eating solid foods beyond my teen years. At the ripe old age of eighteen, I underwent an eight-hour surgery to move my upper jaw up and create a lap joint to my lower jaw to extend it outwards. This resulted in a significant improvement in my bite and a large reduction in my jaw pain.

Knowing that the surgery was going to result in weight loss due to my inability to eat, I was aware that I didn't have a buffer of weight to lose.

I worked really hard to gain weight prior to the surgery, eating everything in sight—full-fat milk, donuts, ice cream, high-calorie foods, you name it. I was successful in gaining weight, but what I also accomplished was an unhealthy and unrealistic expectation of what foods I thought I could eat.

After the jaw surgery, I ended up with numerous sinus infections, which led to me being on antibiotics for almost six months straight. I now know that this wiped out all the good bacteria in my gut, which explains why it was the start of many health problems. Over the next few years, I had several staphylococcus infections, fungal infections, gout, recurrent yeast infections, shingles three times, and numerous athletic injuries, including a torn Achilles tendon, not once but twice.

By the time I was in my early twenties, I was overweight, sick, inflamed, and very broken. I had to walk up the stairs sideways because the pain in my knees was so bad I couldn't walk up or down normally. I ended up going to the emergency department several times for severe abdominal pain, with no diagnosis ever determined. I could barely eat anything without severe cramping and was always bloated and gassy. I thought it might be my gallbladder because of the location of most of my pain, but tests always came back negative. I was referred to a rheumatologist and an allergist who both said I was fine. My doctor didn't know what to do with me.

I turned to alternative medicine and forked out thousands of dollars on naturopathic and homeopathic doctors, with some very slow improvements but no major, life-changing results. I was having an emotional breakdown at least a few times each month because I was so overwhelmed and unable to cope. I developed such severe insomnia that I was only sleeping for two to three hours a night, which was often interrupted. I was caught in a bottomless pit of despair, and at times honestly wanted my life to be ended for me so I wouldn't have to suffer anymore. I prayed that I would get hit by a bus or never wake up. I prayed for a miracle cure. I took up meditation, qi gong, acupuncture, and BodyTalk sessions. I dabbled with different diets, trying the "Eat for Your Blood Type" diet, going gluten-free, going vegetarian, and eliminating nightshades, all at

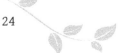

different times. I found out I've been sensitive to food dyes my entire life (hence the childhood temper tantrums) and am lactose intolerant and extremely gluten intolerant. Despite knowing this, nothing changed. So I gave up.

I know what it feels like to be "broken" and to feel like no one understands your pain, discomfort, and irrational, moody thoughts because your body is so out of sorts that you have nothing else to do but cry. After feeling sorry for myself for a good, long time, I would often joke about trying a strict diet of Twinkies and tequila. I figured that since nothing else was working and I felt like garbage all the time, I might as well eat some foods that were fun.

So how did it all change, you might ask? Very slowly, and with a lot of persistence and determination to turn my life around. I was in my early twenties and far too young to accept defeat. Good thing I'm stubborn.

Many years later, I'm now mostly pain-free, sleep much better, and have far more balanced moods. I still have some challenges and some ups and downs just like everyone else, but as a whole, I have taken back my life and my health. In this book, you will find information to educate you on nutrition, exercise, sleep, and stress management to bring some wholeness back to your life. I will teach you how to start with simple changes that you can progress as you achieve success in order to transform your life and reclaim your health.

I truly get what it's like to struggle with your health, and I want you to know that you aren't alone. You don't have to feel that way! To hear more about my story and how I overcame feelings of being broken, check out a bonus video filmed just for you, available at www.yourlifestylestrategy. com/bookbonus.

Chapter One

Start with a Solid
Foundation

ou don't quite know when it happened. Your health has slowly been slipping away. You used to be super healthy and active, and you thought that you were still doing the right things, yet your doctor doesn't agree. They've told you to lose some weight. Your blood pressure or your blood sugars are creeping up, even though you have lots of healthy habits. Sleep isn't as restful as it used to be, and you need to get up to pee at least one time a night. Things just seem out of balance, and you feel like you're broken.

You keep trying different diets with mixed results. Either you're starving yourself to lose weight or not making progress at all. Your lab values haven't budged, and it's stressing you out. Even though you keep trying new things, you see little change. You don't want to become diabetic like your dad because you've seen where that leads, and you don't want to gain that post-menopausal weight that your mom did. It's time to do something now, but you aren't sure where to start.

Your *lifestyle strategy* includes all the habits you are doing to get healthier, plus so much more. It's making the choice to be a healthier version of yourself, along with taking charge of your own health and directing your own medical care. It's preventing problems and diseases so you don't have to undergo unnecessary medical procedures or spend excessive amounts of money to try to regain your health. Your lifestyle strategy is to be intentional in your choices and to look at the implications of your decisions. It's feeling your best and living life to its fullest. It's a lifestyle!

My mission is to empower as many people as I can to be proactive with their health. I want you to achieve optimal health and to be the best that you can be, whatever that looks like—to avoid chronic diseases that you *don't have to get* just because your parents had them. I want you to understand that just because things are common with age (like weight gain, multiple medications, or sleepless nights), it doesn't mean that they are normal or that you need to accept them. The suggestions in this book are for anyone looking to live an optimal life of health and happiness.

Your health begins with a balance between the four pillars of sleep, nutrition, exercise, and mental health. They are all important for maintaining a stable foundation of optimal health. Just like a table, it's ideal to have four legs to have a strong base of support. If you don't have those four pillars in balance, things start to get a little wobbly.

I'm sure you've sat at a table that isn't very stable. Perhaps the ground is a bit uneven or one table leg is a smidge shorter than another. What do you do? Grab a few coasters or a few napkins, fold them up, and tuck them underneath the short table leg, which often does a really good job of balancing the table. The napkins do the job for a while, until they get nudged loose or turn to mush when the floors are washed. They are only a short-term solution.

With your health, taking a medication for something that's preventable is equivalent to napkins under a table leg. So is going on a crash diet or meditating for a few weeks or creating some other good habits. They are short-term, Band-Aid solutions. What happens when that table leg gets even more imbalanced or even knocked out of place? I'm sure you've seen tables with three legs set up as tripods. They can be quite sturdy, but they don't have that same balance and structure as a four-legged

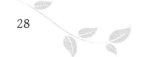

table—they are less forgiving if something happens to alter one of the remaining legs.

That type of "three-legged" scenario happens when aspects of your life get out of balance. Perhaps you are a new mom with a brand new baby at home that's waking you up six or eight or maybe even ten times each night. Your pillar of sleep has just been decimated. It's completely missing or at least hacked off in the middle. You're simply not getting enough sleep.

Or maybe you just found out that you have Crohn's disease and have no idea what to eat. Your nutrition is an absolute disaster, and anything that you put in your body makes you have gas, bloating, or diarrhea. You've been living on bread, white rice, and chicken for weeks and are scared to introduce other foods because it might cause more symptoms to flare up. Your nutrition is in shambles.

The four pillars of health are critical to creating balance in your life. When two or more are out of balance, your entire health collapses. Your goal should be to create the strongest four-legged table you can, to help make you more resilient to whatever life throws at you. And it will. There's always something that's going to pop up. Life likes to throw you curveballs!

A table isn't complete based solely on the state of its *legs* (pillars). It needs a strong top to hold everything together. That's where your digestion comes in. The four key pillars set the foundation for your digestion. At the same time, your digestion sets the foundation for the four pillars. You can't have one without the other.

On top of your table are two other factors that can vary dramatically depending on your unique situation. They are your lifestyle factors and medical conditions. Some people have very little to worry about in these areas, while others were dealt a poor hand and have lots to deal with.

Base these two components on a shaky or uneven table, and what do you think will happen to them? They won't stand a chance. If you have diabetes and you're trying to manage it with medications alone, it may not be enough. You might be able to get away with poor lifestyle habits for a little while, but the progression of your diabetes might happen faster than it would with a solid foundation of healthy habits.

A tabletop without legs is just a slab of wood. The legs without a top are just pretty dowels. Together, they create something beautiful.

The Bucket Analogy

You've probably heard the saying, "it's the straw that broke the camel's back." Your health is kind of the same way. I like to compare health to a bucket full of water. It's the little stuff that often breaks your *table* or makes your *bucket* overflow.

Unfortunately, you can't easily see how much water is in your bucket. You also can't easily know if you have a big bucket or a little one. Many factors add stuff to your bucket. That's what I call it: *stuff*. Because we all have *stuff* that happens to us. It's not that you're broken or bad or doing things wrong. It's just *stuff*. Under the surface, without even realizing it, your problem has been growing or brewing for months or years because of the *stuff* going on in your life.

Some of your stuff might include having poor posture for your entire life or poor ergonomics at your job. Those incorrect postures, over time, wear on your body and create imbalances, tight spots, tension, and eventually, pain and injury. But they don't just happen overnight. Other stuff might be emotional, such as being stressed at work, juggling too many balls at one time, or not sleeping enough.

Your genetics determine the size of your bucket and how much of a buffer you have to handle all the stuff life throws at you. It's how much room you have to tolerate additional stressors. Some of us are blessed with really good genes and can handle lots of stuff. That's the person who can eat whatever they want and not gain weight. They can drink a cup of coffee and go straight to bed. Some of us got the short end of the genetic stick. We have really small buckets with little room as a buffer.

The way a traditional health care system works is that you don't go to see your health care professional until your bucket overflows. That's

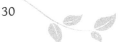

when you actually develop symptoms or chronic issues that are difficult to get rid of. You might wonder where they came from. How did this *suddenly* happen?

Your bucket might overflow from a huge, traumatic event—a death in the family, an injury, or a heart attack. It forces a giant tsunami to come roaring out of your bucket. Your world suddenly crumbles, leaving you unsure of what happened. Other times, your bucket overflows much more slowly, from a small ripple. That's the *straw* on poor Alice the Camel's back.

If you know anything about fluid mechanics, you probably know more than me! But stay with me—it will all become clear in a moment. What I *do* know about the water in your bucket is that it has a meniscus. That's the adhesion that holds that bulb of water above the rim of your bucket. You can keep adding more water above the rim without it overflowing, but only for so long. Once you have too much surface tension, caused by a tiny ripple or just a little too much water, it overflows—maybe not a lot, but it starts to drip a little. That's how some health issues appear. In small trickles.

That's when you typically respond to an issue. You go see your doctor to treat your lower back injury. You see your dentist for that tender spot just under the gums. You mop up the water that's making the floor slippery around your bucket. But you don't dump out the bucket. You never look into the *cause* of your issue. You treat the symptoms.

What you *need* to do is dump out your bucket, get rid of all the *stuff* that's accumulated over your lifetime, and start again. Then you want to start to prevent more stuff from going into your bucket in the first place. Now, that's easier said than done.

The following chapters will give you tools and strategies to empty your bucket and prevent it from filling again. This book will teach you how to manage each of the seven factors (sleep, nutrition, exercise, mental health, digestion, lifestyle conditions, and medical factors) to the best of your abilities. When all of these areas are in balance, you are able to achieve optimal health, or at least get closer to it than you are now.

Understanding Health and Wellness

Between 75 and 80 percent of health care budgets are spent treating preventable chronic diseases. When you look at the time that we as health care professionals spend with patients, about 80 percent of our time is spent taking care of only 20 percent of patients. It doesn't take a rocket scientist to understand that this model isn't sustainable.

It shouldn't be alarming to you that rates of chronic diseases are going up. It's plastered all over the media and attached to many different social issues. By 2030, it is estimated that 171 million US citizens will be diagnosed with various chronic diseases. Think of the financial impact on the economy! Canada and the United Kingdom aren't all that far behind—just give us a bit more time, and we'll hit those numbers, too. To make matters worse, smoking, unhealthy diet, physical activity, and problem drinking make up 38 percent of all deaths in the United States. These habits are completely modifiable. That means that almost 40 percent of *all deaths* are *preventable.*

It's pretty scary to think that two out of every five people die for no good reason. Reversing this process and starting to focus on prevention *before* things start to go awry will go a long way in reducing health care costs and cutting down on chronic diseases. In the United States, it is estimated that by addressing the modifiable risk factors for chronic diseases, almost $500 billion could be saved per year. Other nations present similar statistics. Some sources even suggest that for every one dollar invested in disease prevention programs, we are able to save five dollars in treatment costs. That seems like a pretty good return on investment to me. But making these changes requires a paradigm shift both for health care professionals and the general public, which is on the cusp of happening.

As patients, we need to take responsibility for our own personal health and start implementing habits that help us to maintain a healthy weight, control our blood sugar and stress levels, and sleep more. We need to stop comparing ourselves to the average person because average is no longer healthy. We need to stop blaming other people for why we have problems and take responsibility for our own actions.

For those of us who are health care professionals, we need to be more assertive with our patients and identify when their lab work is starting to move outside of the normal range, in order to address chronic diseases before they become full-blown and it's too late to reverse symptoms. We need to push for funding to be directed to programs focused on prevention. And we need to push for disease prevention techniques as a mandatory part of our education.

However, these two changes rely on a couple of things: time and money! As I mentioned, our current health care model spends most of its budget on treating acute symptoms, with most medical care being performed in hospitals or clinics. Health care professionals are overwhelmed with long waiting lists and have so many other things that they need to do that there simply isn't enough time in the day to focus on prevention.

The Foundation of Health

Ask any good nurse who they learned about most in school, and they'll likely mention the pioneer Florence Nightingale. She was a nurse who lived from 1820–1910 and advocated the concept that "prevention is better than curing." At the time, this concept sounded crazy and was difficult to convince people to buy into. Patients were dying from infections in the hospital or suffering through long recovery times, and Florence saw key areas for possible change. She advocated for several canons: key components that were essential for patients to recover from illness. They included essentials we follow today such as food, ventilation, light, noise, cleanliness/hygiene, variety, and hope.

While these canons are much more recognized today, we still have a long way to go to fully integrate them to increase the health of our population. The concept of integrating wholesome nutrition, stress management, better sleep, or exercise into our medical programs makes sense but is rarely executed. Some of these components exist in medical programs or when patients are hospitalized, but they are often considered an afterthought. Rather than relying on medical programs or teams to implement these components for you, it's time to start taking charge of your own health.

Before we get into the nitty-gritty details of how to be a more active player in your long-term health, it is important to clarify a few terms, just to make sure that we are on the same page. It's pretty easy for me to sling around terms such as *health* or *optimal health* and assume that you know what I'm talking about. It is another thing altogether to have a consensus of what those terms mean. I know, through my years of experience working in the health and fitness industries, that there is no one clear definition for either of those terms, so I'll try to help provide you with a better idea of what each of them means.

Health

One of the most common definitions of health is *the absence of disease*. I strongly believe that being healthy should be more than just not being sick. If you are simply existing between periods of sickness, that's a pretty sad balance in life, and it's far from health.

Merriam-Webster's Dictionary covers this same concept in part 1a of their definition, defining *health* as: "freedom from physical disease or pain." However, they go on to add in part 1b: "the general condition of the body." I agree with this aspect of their definition, in that we aren't just looking at one particular component to define health; it's how everything is working together. Just because one part of the body is healthy, it doesn't mean the whole body is. We should also look outside the physical body and assess the health of our mental state, as that interacts with our physical health.

Although Wikipedia is not a highly credible source for complex topics, I like part of their definition of health, because it makes it more approachable. They define health as: "a level of functional and/or metabolic efficiency of an organism, often implicitly human." This definition points to efficiency—how well things are working in the system. Our bodies are complex systems that need to work well in order to be healthy. Makes sense, right? So let's agree that health is *efficiency and balance* between the complex interactions of our body systems, along with the absence of disease or pain.

Optimal Health

To add an additional component to the concept of health, Merriam-Webster's Dictionary adds part **2a to its definition:** "flourishing condition." Isn't that what you should be doing when you are healthy—flourishing?

Are you truly flourishing? Most of the clients I've worked with would agree that they are not flourishing. Some of them are just getting by, coasting, or making do with what they've got. Is that really what you want for your health? To just settle for average? I want you to have so much more than that. I want you to achieve optimal health.

Many sources describe optimal health as "complete well-being" or a balance between the components of health: physical, emotional, spiritual, social, and intellectual. It's more than just athletic performance, body composition, skin health, the absence of disease, or mental or physical components, but rather, a combination of all of these. It's being able to maintain vigor with age and having a high quality of life along the way.

It's important to note that optimal health is not a static point where, once you achieve it, you'll always be there. Optimal health will ebb and flow depending on your life circumstances. I'd suggest that "optimal health" is what's optimal for you right now—in this situation, with your own circumstances taken into account. Your optimal health during a stressful time in life is going to look dramatically different than your optimal health while you're on vacation.

Rather than chasing an endpoint that will never be reached, I want you to think about how you can be the healthiest version of you in this moment. Not a year from now, not five years from now. Right now! With all the *stuff* going on in your life. Because it's just *stuff*. Your stuff could be work stress, busy kids' schedules, Christmas holidays, a vacation, a sick family member, an injury, whatever. There will always be *stuff*, so accept that and start making better choices today. Make your lifestyle choices in line with being the best, healthiest version of yourself today (whatever day that is), and you'll be on the road to optimal health.

To motivate you even more, Michael P. O'Donnell suggests tying together your core passions and optimal health. What does that mean? Identify what you *love* to do and figure out how being healthier will help you do it better, longer, or faster, depending on what it is. Once you understand how being healthy allows you to enjoy more of the things you love, you'll be more motivated to make choices that keep you healthy. Sounds simple, doesn't it? It is!

Let's move on to explore some specifics of how you can strive for your *optimal* level in those seven key pillars of your health.

Pillar 1: Sleep

"If you have difficulty sleeping or are not getting enough sleep of good quality, you need to learn the basics of sleep hygiene, make appropriate changes, and possibly consult a sleep expert."

—ANDREW WEIL

"Sleep is that golden chain that ties our health and our bodies together."

—THOMAS DEKKER

"For there is nothing quite so terror-inducing as the loss of sleep. It creates phantoms and doubts, causes one to question one's own abilities and judgment, and, over time, dismantles from within, the body."

—CHARLIE HUSTON, *SLEEPLESS*

Chapter Two

Why Do We Sleep?

S leep involves anatomical structures, biochemical pathways, and biological processes. That's a whole lot of technical information, so let's just understand that sleep involves an interaction between environmental influences and your specific health history.

Sleep is made up of two key dimensions: depth (quality) and duration (quantity). Sleep operates on various levels of very complex architecture. You've probably heard of delta sleep or theta sleep. I could spend countless hours talking about the different sleep stages (although I'd probably bore myself). But all you need to know is that there are different stages of sleep when the brain operates at different levels (hertz), and the brain cycles through these stages several times throughout the night. Improving my sleep quality dramatically changed my life.

My Sleepless Nights

Growing up, I was always a poor sleeper. I had a hard time falling asleep and staying asleep. Once I was asleep, I had disturbing nightmares that woke me up in a cold sweat, and I was unable to shake their memories in order to fall back asleep. I would dream the same terrifying dreams night after night, sometimes several times in the same night.

As I got older, my sleep quality got worse. By the time I reached my early twenties, I was only sleeping about two to three hours each night over the course of a six to eight-hour span. I literally thought I was going crazy. I thought that I might have schizophrenia or bipolar disorder because I kept having such irrational thoughts and mood swings, not understanding where these thoughts were coming from.

Eventually, I got assessed through a program that quickly identified that I was not actually going crazy (although I felt like I was). I just needed more sleep. I got referred to a sleep program in the hospital and started working with a qualified sleep professional.

She literally saved my life.

It wasn't always easy or fun. I remember many sleepless nights sitting alone on my sofa trying to implement "calming techniques" so that I could get some sleep before the next day. I remember keeping sleep logs, feeling overwhelmed, alone, and hopeless, thinking that it would never get better. But little by little, it did. By going through sleep assessment and different types of sleep therapy, I was able to retrain my brain and body into relearning what sleep was, and I gradually improved my sleep quality. After lots of consistency and hard work, I'm now able to get seven to nine hours of consolidated sleep almost every night. I have more energy, can think clearly, and am no longer a volatile ticking time bomb about to explode.

I want you to feel this same sense of control over your own sleep and to be able to reap the health benefits that only a good night's sleep can provide. This chapter will help outline some of the basic principles around sleep and give you some strategies you can easily implement in your life.

Before we jump too far down the rabbit hole, it's critical that we understand what makes us want to sleep. We have two different processes that make sleep happen. The first process is called *sleep drive* or *sleep pressure*. Sleep drive is the internal signal that yells at you, "go to sleep now!" making your eyelids droopy, making your head bob, and causing you to fall asleep in front of the television even though your bed is just upstairs. Sleep drive increases between each period of sleep and then is relieved or decreased by sleeping. When the sleep drive mechanism is working properly, you'll wake up in the morning and start building this drive up as the day progresses. By the time your normal bedtime comes around, about sixteen hours later, sleep drive is at its peak, providing extremely strong cues that it's time to go to sleep. Then you fall asleep, and this process starts all over again the next day.

The other process occurs in a more rhythmic pattern independent of sleep. This master conductor or circadian clock in the brain (specifically, the suprachiasmatic nucleus—say that three times fast!) will respond to environmental cues such as sunlight or bright light exposure. When operating normally, this process tells the body, "Hey, it's bright outside, time to get up," or, "It's been dark for a while, you should go to sleep."

Unfortunately, in today's modern society, we have royally messed up both of these processes, so our bodies are getting mixed-up cues. We spend long hours under bright lights at work and are constantly tuned into our smartphones and laptops, giving our brains the signal that it's time to be awake when it really isn't. Once this internal clock gets messed up, we shift our sleep cycles because we aren't tired, making this even worse. To complicate it, we try to catch up on sleep on weekends by sleeping in, which messes this up even further. No wonder there are so many people who have insomnia and other sleep issues!

These issues don't get fixed overnight or even in one or two nights. If your sleep issue is short-lived, the treatment will likely be effective in a much shorter period of time. Generally, improving sleep issues takes time and consistent patterning to reprogram the brain regarding what it should do.

The trick to improving sleep is consistency! You will need to stick to habits for weeks or months, and—for some of you—potentially for years, if you've been dealing with sleeping difficulties your entire life. Now, that sounds discouraging, doesn't it? But it doesn't have to be. Essentially, the longer you've had sleeping difficulties, the longer it will likely take to correct them. There's no magic bullet to fix your sleep overnight. If you've had sleep issues for twenty years, what's another year to get it fixed? You'll be glad you invested the time when you are able to wake up feeling more refreshed and well rested.

Why We Sleep

Sleep fulfills three key functions that help keep our bodies in check. The first is energy conservation (savings), where our metabolism is regulated and energy homeostasis (balance) occurs.

The second function is to consolidate (pull together) our memories, where they are encoded in a part of the brain called the hippocampus (not to be confused with the hippopotamus—they are *very* different). Despite being a small part of the brain, the hippocampus has a big role in turning short-term memories into long-term memories.

The final function of sleep is to suppress primitive behaviors like eating, sex, aggression, and movement. For example, if you started reacting to your dreams, swinging your arms or legs around, your partner sleeping next to you would likely get hurt. Likewise, you don't want to be eating in the middle of the night while you're asleep, or you might end up gaining a lot of weight. In some people, the part of the brain that suppresses these types of behaviors can get messed up, resulting in inappropriate behaviors when they sleep. That's when a sleep specialist is required!

The restorative theory of sleep proposes that sleep is also a way of restoring the body back to the best version of itself so that we feel refreshed in the morning. Sleep helps restore hormone levels, the immune system, chemical messengers, and brain and nerve intersections. Chemicals, hormones, and neurotoxins that build up during the day are cleared out of the body at night. Growth hormone secretion should peak during sleep, which is also a part of this restoration process.

How Much Sleep Do You Need?

After reviewing multiple studies on what *optimal sleep* looks like, I've found that most experts agree that the duration should be somewhere between seven to nine hours of sleep for adults. This does vary a bit; anywhere from six hours to ten hours was listed. Both the American Academy of Sleep Medicine and the Sleep Research Society state that adults should

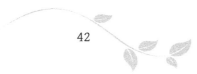

get seven or more hours of sleep per night on a regular basis to promote optimal health.

The problem with offering a range of recommendations is that nine times out of ten, you will self-select the lower end. Just because you *want* to sleep less doesn't mean you should. The other caveat to these recommendations is that the sleep time should be preceded by proper sleep hygiene, consolidated (all together, with no waking up), and follow a consistent sleep pattern or architecture, hitting all the proper levels of sleep required for recovery.

Is it possible to sleep eight hours or more each night and still be sleep deprived? As few as five mini awakenings (micro-arousals) per hour of sleep can result in daytime sleepiness and decreases in performance. Micro-arousals can be so tiny that you actually have no idea that they are happening, but you wake up feeling exhausted, even though you think you slept through the entire night.

"But I Can Function Just Fine on Less than Seven Hours of Sleep"

Nick was a big-city police officer with fourteen years on the job. He was a highly driven kind of guy, always wanting to do more. He joined his local union and eventually became the local president, taking on much more work and responsibility on top of his normal shifts. He lived on an acreage and had a family with three kids who were busy in many activities, making it difficult to coordinate driving schedules with his wife. Nick wanted more fulfillment in his life, so he also volunteered for a few local charities a few times each year.

Nick liked to be busy and had a hard time saying no to anything that sounded interesting. Being a police officer with a physically demanding job, Nick worked hard to maintain his fitness, working out when he could and eating relatively healthy. Due to his rotating-shift work schedule, Nick's sleep wasn't ideal even at the best of times. He thrived on adrenaline and bragged to his co-workers about how little sleep he could get away with. Nick commented that he felt even better with four hours of sleep than he normally did with six hours, and was able to get so much more done.

Stories like Nick's are incredibly common. Many people feel they perform better when they get fewer hours of sleep. Unfortunately, despite feeling like we are able to perform better, we are actually so hopped up on adrenaline that we don't realize how sleep deprived we are.

The problem with assessing our own level of function is that we aren't aware of our own level of cognitive impairment. We adapt to this decrease in sleep quickly but are far from functioning at an optimal level. It's sort of like being a functional alcoholic who's able to have a few drinks in their system and still perform normal tasks without appearing impaired. In the case of sleep deprivation, you are a **functioning-sleep-deficit-aholic**, walking around thinking you are doing just fine.

This is arguably one of the most important points in the field of sleep research. We don't know that we need more sleep because the body is so good at accommodating this change. This accommodation is meant as a short-term adaptation to lack of sleep, not as a long-term lifestyle habit.

Need more concrete examples? Countless studies have been done on hospital residency programs—one of the most chronically sleep-deprived groups. In one such study, one group of interns were given a traditional schedule. Another group was given a modified schedule that included more hours of sleep. Interns who worked the traditional schedule made **36 percent more serious medical errors** and had **more than twice the rate of attention mistakes** than interns who worked under the modified schedule. Now, I don't know about you, but if I had the choice of which doctor was working on me, I'd definitely opt for the physician on the modified schedule!

Your job may or may not be as critical as a medical intern, but I'll bet that when you're sleep deprived, your risk for errors would rate around the same. How would you feel about making 36 percent more serious errors in your job? Or losing focus twice as often? How productive would you be in your day? There's a pretty good chance you'd be missing out on key business opportunities.

Let's say you are only a little sleep deprived and could benefit from a 10 percent increase in performance. Take a peek at your job metrics and see what a 10 percent increase could do for you. Ten percent could

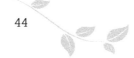

mean more clients or an increase in your salary. It could mean that you're more efficient and have 10 percent more time to go do the fun things you want to do. That could add up to a lot of change over the course of a year or a decade.

Many people are sleep deprived because of the demands of their work, family, or social responsibilities, and from existing sleep disorders. Other factors that affect sleep are medical conditions that require medications that disturb sleep, or injuries/pain that make a normal sleep cycle almost impossible. Sleep deprivation also has many mental, physiological, emotional, social, and work-related effects, as listed in the chart below.

Mental Effects	<ul><li>Cognitive/behavioral performance</li><li>Alertness: sleepiness, fatigue, tension, and lack of vigilance, attention, and focus</li><li>Judgment: confusion, problems with logic and reasoning</li><li>Analysis: difficulties with flexible thinking and complex mathematical tasks</li></ul>
Physiological Effects	<ul><li>Insulin Resistance</li><li>Metabolic dysregulation</li><li>Gastrointestinal problems</li><li>Cardiovascular problems</li><li>Shortness of breath</li><li>Increased heart rate/blood pressure</li><li>Increased sympathetic nervous system activity</li><li>Neural changes</li></ul>
Emotional Effects	<ul><li>Depression, fatigue</li><li>Anxiety, irritability</li><li>Decreased libido</li><li>Increased perception of pain</li><li>Increased emotional burden</li><li>Decreased quality of life</li></ul>

Social Effects	▶ Decrease in pleasurable activities
	▶ Lack of energy to participate in pleasurable activities
	▶ Marital conflict
	▶ Drowsiness at inappropriate times
Work Effects	▶ Increased absenteeism
	▶ Increased errors or accidents
	▶ Unplanned drowsiness/naps (may cause tension, embarrassment)
	▶ Denied advancement, reprimanded, fired
	▶ Increased health-related consequences

Looking at this massive list of consequences of poor sleep, it's hard to ignore the impact of sleep on our health. *All* of these side effects can be linked to lack of sleep or poor quality sleep—you don't have to have insomnia or other sleep disorders to have these side effects.

Focusing on sleep may be an easy place to start to improve your health and may fix more issues than you even intended. If your aim is to create a solid foundation of health, it's hard to go wrong by addressing your sleep quality and quantity.

In addition to the long list of consequences of unhealthy sleep habits, you are also putting yourself at risk for:

- Breast cancer
- Cardiovascular disease
- Coronary heart disease/coronary artery calcification
- Type two diabetes
- Hypertension
- Inflammation
- Obesity
- Heart attack
- Stroke

What's most interesting about this list is that many if not all of these chronic diseases are preventable! You've probably heard the complaints about how expensive these diseases are to treat and how much time they

take to treat. Yet if we spent more time on prevention, it would be a completely different story. By working to improve your sleep, you are decreasing the risk of these common and costly diseases and opening yourself to a plethora of other health benefits.

Factors Affecting Sleep

You are super busy just like me. You're on the go all day and want to come home to get a good night's sleep before doing it all over again the next day. I often hear about how poorly people sleep, yet they overlook all of the factors that affect their sleep quality and quantity, such as:

- Time of day/circadian rhythm (internal and external cues for sleep)
- Light exposure (during the day and prior to sleep)
- Preceding waking duration (how long they've been awake, sleep deprivation)
- Previous activity
- Room temperature
- Caffeine/nicotine/alcohol (stimulants/sedatives)
- Medications
- Sleep history—days/weeks/months
- Medical conditions/injuries (chronic obstructive pulmonary disease, hypoglycemia, gastroesophageal reflux, congestive heart failure, renal disease, neurologic issues: head trauma, brain tumor, encephalitis, etc.)
- Fever or other illnesses

You may also notice a disruption in your sleep patterns if you have poor sleep hygiene or are deprived of sleep for various reasons. Temporary circadian rhythm disturbances, such as jet lag, and prolonged changes to sleep cycles, such as shift work, can change sleep quality. Emotional stress may also be a factor in sleeping too much or too little. In the next chapter, Sleep Essentials, we'll go into more detail about the factors that affect sleep and how you can improve your sleep quality and quantity.

Chapter Three

Sleep Essentials

*C*urrently, our society does not value sleep. Everyone *wants* to be on the latest fad diet, but sleep isn't sexy or catchy in the same way. What is sexy is the ability to "perform well" on as little sleep as possible. This mentality comes from people thinking that they need to get more done in a day, to be tougher, and to see how little sleep they can get away with. It's an all-or-nothing mentality where people think less is more. Very few people are interested in cutting other things out of their day in order to get more sleep. This approach is definitely not working, and something needs to change.

Sleep experts agree that it is important to educate the public and health care professionals on the benefits of optimal sleep. They want to encourage adults to get adequate sleep and to promote awareness of the role of sleep on health. They also want to understand the economic and social benefits of getting adequate sleep, as this area is poorly understood.

Sleep itself is a huge issue in society. Between one-third and two-thirds of North Americans have sleeping problems, and as we get older, about 58 percent of older adults report having sleeping difficulties. Ten to fifteen percent of people report that their insomnia is severe enough to impair daytime functioning. That's a lot of people affected by poor sleep! Insomnia symptoms can include difficulty initiating or maintaining sleep and/or waking too early in the morning, accompanied by daytime dysfunction, which occurs in about 25 to 30 percent of adults.

The takeaway of all this is that we as a society are not getting enough sleep. This is a huge issue, and we need to address this now. So, how do we start? When it comes to sleep, it's important to begin by determining how to meet your essential physiological needs.

Maslow's hierarchy of needs shows that our physiological needs are at the bottom of the pyramid. These are the essential needs that we *must* meet in order to survive. Physiological needs include breathing, water, food, **sleep**, shelter, and clothing. Sleep is often overlooked, but it is **not** an option. You **need** to have it, and you need to start prioritizing it.

The next level of Maslow's hierarchy of needs is security, which is also often overlooked when considering sleep needs. If you are not in a safe and secure environment, you'll be unable to meet your sleep needs to have a proper, restful sleep.

Jerry came into my office well dressed. He was clean and presented just as typically as any other patient I've seen. Jerry presented with chronic pain and had very poor sleep, getting only about three to four hours of interrupted sleep a night. He supplemented with naps between one to three hours long in the afternoon just to get by.

Jerry's pain originally started from a back injury at work, and he ended up on long-term disability, living in low-income housing. After inquiring more about Jerry's situation, I was able to find out that his poor sleep was because his building had a bedbug infestation, and the manager had pulled all of the mattresses so that the building could be fumigated. Jerry had been sleeping on either the floor or his rickety old sofa for months because he wasn't able to afford a new bed. At that point, he also wasn't able to bring a new piece of furniture into the building because of the bedbugs. Had I not done further investigations regarding Jerry's safety and security, I may never have discovered why he was sleeping poorly.

If you are having difficulty meeting your essential needs, there are resources out there to help you, such as social workers, subsidized housing programs, or getting set up with income funding such as Worker's

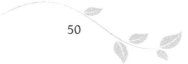

Compensation, unemployment earnings, or other options in your area. There are also safe housing programs that are available, in which rental units must meet certain safety standards such as being up to fire codes, being free of bugs, having windows and doors that lock, and offering safe air conditioning or heating that actually works. It's shocking that we even need to think about this, but I've had patients living in substandard living situations. I'm sure you know people in similar situations.

You'll also want to make sure that you are in a safe situation where you're not worried about concerns of abuse that will keep you up at night, sleeping with "one eye open," so to speak. Certain risk factors that put you in a vulnerable population include your race, gender, age, disability, income, and sexual orientation. You're also considered vulnerable if you don't have your own living space at the moment—in other words, if you are technically homeless. This may be a temporary measure, such as a period of time when you are living with friends until a new house is built, or you may perpetually be in a vulnerable position.

People who are part of a vulnerable or homeless population often don't consider themselves vulnerable. They will commonly use statements like, "I'm just staying with family or friends for now," or, "my situation is temporary," without recognizing that that actually means they are in a vulnerable position.

Sleep is one of the fundamental components of meeting our physiological needs. You'll want to consider some specific questions about your current sleeping situation. Here are some examples of questions for you to determine whether you are part of a vulnerable population.

General Questions

Do you have a home or a consistent place to sleep?

Many people may not consider themselves homeless but may not have a consistent place to sleep. Having a regular place to call "home" is key to creating a solid foundation for sleep. If you do not have a consistent place to sleep and are not currently working on improving this situation, consider connecting with a social worker or other sources of support to help gain this security.

Do you have your own bed? Do you share your bed? (e.g., partners, kids, pets). Is this disruptive to you? Or comforting?

Having a consistent bed to sleep in is part of the foundation for improving sleep. In some cultures, it is comforting to have the family sleep together in one bed or on the floor; in other cultures, this is very disruptive. Consider your own cultural preferences. Some people let pets sleep in their beds, which may wake them up throughout the night—if this is the case, the animals should be crated or left in another room overnight. Often, it's the owner who has a more difficult time making this change than the animal! Your health is more important than the habit of letting your animals co-sleep in your bed.

What is the age of your mattress? What is the quality of your mattress?

Mattresses are not built to last forever. In cases where multiple people sleep in a bed or larger dogs sleep in the bed, the mattress will wear out faster than if it's used by just one person. Check the manufacturer's recommendations for ideal replacement. Poorer quality beds will need to be replaced more often. Replace mattresses that are sagging, have springs poking out, and are visibly soiled or damaged.

Are you able to control the temperature in your room? Is your room too hot or cold? Are you able to pay for appropriate heating/cooling?

It is important to sleep in an environment that is not too hot or too cold. If you are unable to afford the cost of heating/cooling your house, you'll want to connect with someone who can help improve your financial security.

Safety and Security

Do you have any safety concerns in your home?

Domestic violence is a huge concern for many women, men, and children. What is your risk of domestic violence? If you do have safety concerns for you or your family, consult with a qualified professional to help you sort out this challenging situation.

Do you have any concerns over losing your house? Or your current bed?

People who have no set place to sleep, are living paycheck to paycheck, or are at high risk of losing their home are more prone to experiencing disrupted sleep. Increased stress or uncertainty can lead to sleeplessness and insomnia, and can possibly progress to other negative coping skills such as alcohol and drug use. If you have any financial concerns, seek out assistance to improve your financial situation.

Cleanliness

Is your bed/mattress free of bed bugs, urine, other stains/contaminants? Are you able to wash your sheets on a regular basis?

These questions likely seem offensive, especially if you are living in a stable situation. However, this is an important concern that should be addressed. I've worked with clients who dress well, smell clean, and would appear put together but are living in substandard housing with bed bug infestations and no ability to wash bulky items like sheets and blankets.

Chapter Four

Evaluating Sleep

By now, you are probably starting to realize that it would be beneficial to evaluate your sleep in more detail, but you may not know how. You can start by keeping a detailed sleep log that tracks your sleep time, sleep problems, and subjective sleep quality.

Sleep logs are readily available online, and I've also attached one in the appendix section that you can photocopy. Sleep logs can vary dramatically in the details that they record. Ideally, you'll want to use one that records specific details about sleep, as that is more informative to identify when you are having difficulty sleeping.

Let's explore how to use a sleep log!

Sample Sleep Log:

Row A: Record if you had any naps and the total minutes that you slept.

Rows B and C: will identify any stimulants or depressants that may affect sleep, along with medications and supplements used.

Row D: the time that you went to bed with the intention or goal of sleeping.

Row E: accounts for time awake in bed prior to the intention of sleep. In this time, you may be reading, watching TV, or doing other activities. (In the next section, on sleep hygiene, we'll discuss how to reduce

		Day 1	Day 2	Day 3	Day 4	Day 5	Day 6	Day 7
A	I napped for (xxx) minutes yesterday:	0	0	0	0	0	0	0
B	Sleep aids I took last night:	5mg Melatonin, 350mg Magnesium	5mg Melatonin, 350mg Magnesium	5mg Zopiclone	0	5mg Melatonin, 350mg Magnesium	5mg Melatonin, 350mg Magnesium	5mg Melatonin, 350mg Magnesium
C	List any caffeine, nicotine, alcohol, drugs consumed today:	1 Glass Red wine	0	0	0	1 Green Tea	0	0
D	I went to bed at (xxx) time:	9:00	10:45	11:00	9:30	9:00	9:15	9:15
E	I turned off the light intending to sleep after (xxx) minutes:	30	45	30	30	45	45	30
F	From the time I started trying to sleep, it took (xxx) minutes to fall asleep:	15	75	30	30	5	30	30
G	My planned wake-up time this morning: (write none if you didn't have one)	none	6:00	7:00	none	7:00	7:00	none
H	My actual final wake-up time this morning: (no more sleep after this)	6:00	6:00	6:45	6:30	7:00	7:00	8:30
I	Time I got out of bed:	7:10	6:00	7:00	6:45	7:05	7:05	8:45
J	"Number of times I woke up in the night: (write ""0"" if you did not wake up)"	3	5	0	0	2	3	1
K	How long, all together, was I awake in the middle of the night? (minutes)	90	140	0	0	90	190	30
L	Total Minutes in Bed Time between D + I	610	435	480	555	610	615	750
M	Total minutes awake (Row E + F + K)	135	260	60	60	140	265	90
N	How many minutes sleep did I get last night? (Row L – Row M) (Goal: 420-540)	475	175	420	495	470	350	660
O	Sleep Efficiency [(Row L-M)/L]x 100= %	78%	40%	88%	89%	77%	57%	88%
P	Quality of sleep: 1=very poor, 10=excellent	8	3	6	7	8	5	6
	Notes:	Feel not bad, still a bit tired, one of my better nights since house sitting	First night at home after house sitting. At hockey game with friends, hard falling asleep, feel more tired today after solid sleep	Hubby out for poker night and got home late, had friend over, Headache on/off all day, feeling tired today	First Day back at school, slight headache today, family stressors-friend injured ankle, cousins in town	Hubby on nights-slept alone	Hubby on nights-slept alone, bath before bed, woke with sore throat, could have gone back to bed at 10am (had to get ready for class)	feeling rundown yesterday-sore throat, much better this morning

or eliminate this time.) This section and below can be filled out the next morning so that it doesn't interfere with falling asleep. You don't need to keep a stopwatch by your bed, as you will get a good sense of time once you start tracking your sleep in detail.

Row F: will tell you how easy or difficult it is to fall asleep. Record the time required to fall asleep here in minutes.

Row G: the time you were planning to get up, or what time the alarm clock was set for.

Row H: the time you actually woke up and did not get any sleep beyond this time.

Row I: the time you actually got out of bed. This time can differ dramatically from the time when you actually woke up.

Row J: the number of times you woke up in the night.

Row K: adds up the total time that you were awake during the night, regardless of the cause.

Row L: totals up the time in bed. This is *not* the time asleep in bed. To get this answer, add Row D + Row I.

Row M: totals up the time awake in bed. To get this answer, add Row E + Row F + Row K.

Row N: gives you the total of how much sleep you got during the night. To get this answer, subtract Row M from Row L. Despite the goal being between 420–540 minutes, the focus should be on improving your sleep quality first, then focusing on your quantity.

Row O: calculates your sleep efficiency or how well you are sleeping. You'll want to consistently have 80 to 85 percent efficiency before you start increasing your sleep time in fifteen-minute increments or less.

Row P: This is where you get to add your personal opinion on the quality of your sleep. You may have a short night of sleep and feel great or have a longer sleep and feel horrible. This section is completely up to how you feel.

Notes: There is room below the chart to make any notes you need to keep track of other things going on in your life that may contribute to a good or bad night's sleep. Taking notes helps to account for important details that may be forgotten later.

Wow! That seems like a lot of stuff to record, and it is, but it all has value for you. Every piece of information tells you where you are struggling with your sleep. Some people have a hard time falling asleep while others have a hard time staying asleep. Tracking lots of different components of sleep will help you pinpoint where you will get your greatest return on your time.

I remember being the patient and having to record my sleep every night. I did this faithfully for several years. Sometimes, I hated doing it. Not because it was time-consuming—it truthfully only takes a few minutes to fill out—but because of the monotony of the task. I wanted to do anything other than track my sleep. At one point, I did have to stop because I became so obsessed with watching the clock and counting the minutes I was awake in bed that I was actually making things worse. Once I was able to stop watching the clock, I was able to resume keeping a sleep log. The value it gave me and my physician was tremendous.

As a patient, I was able to see the gradual improvement in my sleep, which I wouldn't have otherwise noticed. My physician was able to see where I was making improvements and where I was struggling, and then was able to customize the plan based on where I needed the most support. As you work with your sleep log to improve your sleep, please remember that changing sleep habits can take a really long time, especially if you've had sleep issues for years. Be patient and keep at it—the results will be well worth it in the end!

Sleep Hygiene

Have you ever had a tough time getting to sleep because your bed is so full of stuff? Maybe you have a pile of books on your bed or maybe your pets take over so there isn't room for you and your partner to sleep. If this sounds like you, your mind should immediately consider the need to implement sleep hygiene.

Sleep hygiene is a fancy term for a set of guidelines to establish and maintain healthy sleep patterns. It helps set the cues and the clues that

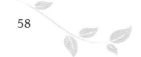

tell the body that it's time to go to bed. It takes a regular, consistent effort to see the benefit from sleep hygiene, which, over time, makes it easier to fall asleep and stay asleep.

If you aren't able to get into bed because there's so much stuff on it, you are setting yourself up for a poor night's sleep and conditioning your body that your bedroom is not a restful, relaxing place to be. With sleep hygiene, you'll learn the importance of consistency and a routine that encourages good sleep habits.

Here are the most common tips and tricks that I've found on sleep hygiene that can help you improve your sleep quality:

Goals for Your Sleep Environment

Make the bedroom pitch black: add black-out blinds, put electrical tape over electronics, put tinfoil on your windows if you have no other options!

> *The darker the better—studies show that even a small amount of light can disrupt sleep patterns.*

Keep the bedroom cool and well ventilated (crack the window).

> *A room that is too hot or too cold can interrupt sleep patterns. Keep the room slightly cool for optimal sleep.*

Reduce excess noise in the sleep environment; some people sleep better with noise, some without. Use earplugs if needed.

> *Some people sleep well with white noise to block out external sounds. Some people need complete silence. This is an area to experiment with!*

The bedroom should only be used for sleep/sex and not for work, watching TV, etc. Remove any of these distractions.

> *Distractions such as work, watching TV, etc., create the association of wakefulness in bed and should be performed outside of the sleep environment and prior to the wind-down period.*

If there is anxiety around sleep, move the alarm clock, wall clock, or watch out of reach so it can't be checked during the night.

> *Moving alarm clocks/watches out of reach prevents you from getting fixated on what time it is if you are awake in the middle of the night.*

Clean up the clutter! Remove anything from the bedroom that isn't absolutely necessary. Keep it neat and tidy to encourage a feeling of relaxation in the bedroom.

> *Keeping a clean room will remove distractions so that you don't get distracted by your "to-do list," and it will create a relaxing environment that will be associated with sleep.*

Have a supportive bed with a level of softness to suit individual needs. Replace the bed and pillow as needed. If you can't remember the last time you bought a new bed, it's time!

> *Having a supportive and comfortable bed is key to a good night's sleep. Get a professional bed fitting to determine what type of mattress will best suit your needs. Mattresses should be rotated according to manufacturers' recommendations to extend their wear. Pillows wear out faster than mattresses and should be replaced more often.*

Goals for Setting a Routine

By consistently going to bed and waking at the same times, you will improve the cueing that you are regularly providing your body. Setting a regular routine also helps hormones work in better balance and become more aligned with their natural "circadian rhythms" (or day/night rotation). Consistency is the name of the game! Establishing optimal hormonal balance takes time and won't change overnight.

People often think that it doesn't matter when they go to bed or wake up. Bodies work best when they follow a normal circadian rhythm, when you go to bed and wake up at the same time each day. By following a

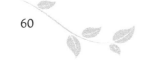

routine on a regular basis, you allow your body to balance the hormones that provide cues that it's time to wake up or time to go to sleep. Start today by planning a set bedtime and wake-up time that fit your schedule.

Go to bed/wake up at the same time every day, regardless of how you slept.

> *This allows for a consistent sleep pattern to be developed. It takes time to be reset and re-established, especially in people who have had no sleep consistency or have had poor sleep habits for years. Initially, you may report difficulty sleeping, especially if you are used to nights with only a few hours of sleep.*

Rather than trying to "catch up" on sleep after a late night, the body responds better to a consistent amount of sleep. Add only a minimal amount of sleep on nights when you need more sleep. If you must "catch up on sleep," add up to a maximum of one hour on either end of your sleep time no more than two days per week.

> *People who sleep for several additional hours on weekends may have difficulty falling asleep on Sunday night because their sleep drive isn't as strong. This then leads to a restless night, less sleep, and waking up on Monday feeling more tired than you did before the weekend.*

Preparing for Sleep

Reduce light exposure, TV, computer, and phone use 90–120 minutes prior to sleep.

> *Light exposure even in tiny amounts will disrupt sleep architecture or duration, as the body receives incorrect cues that it's time to be awake. Using rose-colored lenses or blue blockers prior to bed may significantly improve sleep quality.*

Eliminate caffeine (coffee, tea, chocolate, soft drinks) for at least six hours prior to bed. Avoid smoking prior to going to sleep. Even better—quit smoking.

These stimulants can delay sleep onset or decrease the depth of sleep even without you being aware of this effect. If you claim that you can drink a pot of coffee and then go to sleep, you may fall asleep easily, but you still may not be achieving the optimal sleep depth required for optimal recovery.

Avoid alcohol in the evening and prior to sleep—it affects sleep quality and may cause awakenings during the night.

Alcohol may help you fall asleep faster (or pass out!) but will interfere with the depth of sleep, leading to a choppy or interrupted sleep pattern.

Go to sleep only when drowsy/tired.

This may seem contrary to the advice being given about consistency. If you are going to bed simply because it's bedtime and your mind is spinning from your day, you will likely struggle to fall asleep. Postponing a bedtime until you're drowsy helps you prevent creating a negative association by being restless in bed. If the need to push your bedtime becomes frequent, it's time to rethink sleep habits.

Create a buffer zone—do something calming for 60–90 minutes prior to sleep: yoga, gentle stretching, reading with a dim light, prayer, meditation, listening to calming music, guided relaxation, having a hot bath, etc.

Have you ever been chased by a tiger, then tried to fall asleep right after? This example may be a bit extreme, but essentially, that's what you are doing all day. You end up running around all day long, trying to cram more into the day, and then you wonder why you can't fall asleep the minute your head hits the pillow. The point of a buffer zone is to slow down the mind and cue the body that it's time to sleep. This "wind-down time" lets those stress hormones settle down, letting the body know it's safe to fall asleep.

If you are not able to fall asleep within 15–20 minutes of going to bed or upon waking at night, get out of bed and do a calming activity until you are sleepy.

> Associating a calming activity with sleep will help to teach you the cues needed to recognize that it's time to go to sleep. It doesn't have to be one of the activities listed above, but it should be something that you find enjoyable and relaxing. This is the same strategy to be used if you can't fall asleep or stay asleep. The key, however, is not to engage in a rewarding activity such as watching your favorite TV show or eating, as this encourages disrupted sleep patterns.

Avoid large or heavy meals too close to bed; some people sleep better with some carbohydrates or proteins prior to bed to avoid sugar crashes overnight.

> Dietary needs are different for everyone, so it's difficult to generalize these suggestions. However, literature generally supports smaller meals prior to bedtime. Anyone with blood sugar issues may benefit more from a small protein snack prior to bed to level blood sugars, while others need to boost their blood sugar prior to bed in order to achieve effective sleep.

Interventions

Cognitive behavioral therapy (CBT) may be beneficial for changing thought patterns around sleep.

> Any health care professional can discuss thoughts related to sleep with their patients. I have seen many professionals get positive results by engaging their patients in therapeutic conversations about sleep habits (no additional training required). However, CBT is a specialized competency that requires additional training. The benefit of going through the formal CBT process is that it is well supported in the literature as effective, whereas a therapeutic conversation may not have the same lasting benefits.

For people who have trouble shutting off their brains at night—schedule a regular "thinking time" to come up with your "to-do list" or solve your problems away from bedtime.

> *Keep a journal by your bed or schedule time in the evening to write out your thoughts and worries so you can refer to it the next day.*

Sleep aids:

> **Pharmaceutical** *(e.g., Trazodone, Zopiclone/Imovane, etc.): can be habit-forming—only use these following the advice of a physician, and they are typically indicated as intended for short-term use only.*

> **Natural Remedies** *(e.g., melatonin, 5HTP, Zen Theanine, tryptophan, magnesium, etc.): should be discussed with a physician prior to use to minimize drug interactions/side effects. Natural remedies are not necessarily side effect free and may not be appropriate for use with certain medical conditions.*

> *There are pros/cons to pharmaceutical and natural remedies alike that should be carefully evaluated for each unique situation prior to their use. Discuss options with either a physician or a pharmacist who understands the benefits and risks.*

Ideal Sleep Position

The ideal sleep position is quite controversial. There tends to be a minimal consensus from several research articles that I've read, simply because there are so many variables at play. Some of the factors that you'll want to consider when coming up with an ideal sleeping position are:

- The type of bed and pillows you have
- Your body weight
- Injuries
- Medical conditions

For some good, general sleep recommendations that are applicable to anyone, you'll want to get set up with a good bed system that has a moderate amount of firmness to support your body weight. You will benefit

from a custom fit that is designed specifically for your body shape and weight. Pillows are generally a matter of personal preference and should be replaced when they lose their support and comfort. Pillow choices range from synthetic to down to buckwheat and come in many sizes and varieties of firmness.

The key to a good sleeping position is to maintain a natural, neutral spinal alignment. Ideally, you want to sleep in a level position that supports the natural curvatures of the spine: cervical and lumbar (concave posteriorly/lordosis), and thoracic and sacral (convex posteriorly/kyphosis). Yup, more big words! If that's too much detail and you have no idea what those terms mean, a simple way to evaluate sleep position is to look at what your shoulders and hips are doing. For example, if you prefer sleeping on your side, make sure that your shoulders and hips are stacked directly on top of each other rather than being tilted forward or back, twisting the spine. It's not always necessary to dramatically change your position from where you're currently sleeping; you just want to make sure that you are supported and neutral.

Prioritize your medical conditions, making sure that you are meeting needs for any respiratory symptoms. If you have sleep apnea or any injuries that need to be maintained in a specific position (such as head or back injuries), you'll need to make sure that your sleep position supports these needs. Follow the recommendations of the health care professional who has diagnosed the medical condition. There are likely specific reasons for why you need to sleep in an upright or side position based on complications that may arise if you sleep in an alternative position. Despite wanting to find an *ideal* or *perfect* sleeping position, medical needs always come first.

Although some of these adjusted positions may not create *optimal* sleep, they may need to be used as temporary or permanent positions to prevent further injury or harm. For example, if a supine (back) position is ideal for your spinal alignment but your airway keeps closing in this position, you'll definitely want to adjust to a more upright position. Airway maintenance trumps everything else! For anyone who is at risk of obstructive sleep apnea, you'll want to reduce or completely eliminate back-sleeping.

There are some specific sleep behaviors that tend to be connected with sleeping positions. Poor sleepers tend to change their position more often than those who sleep better. Positions that don't unload the spine, such as sleeping in an upright position, increase spinal fatigue and don't allow the body to fully rest. This is because gravity has a stronger effect on the spine when it's upright than when it's horizontal.

A lying position also allows nourishing spinal fluid to move into places along the spine that are usually compressed during the day, ultimately helping to keep tissues healthy. If you have an injury that forces you to sleep in an upright position, you should use pillows or props to help support your spine so that your spine can unload at least to some degree during the night.

Fatigue

Fatigue can result when you are not getting the right balance between quality or quantity of sleep. Your quality of sleep goes down when you wake up at night or have fragmented sleep. Your total sleep time can be reduced due to work or family responsibilities, illness or injury, stress, or multiple other factors.

Fatigue is considered a perceived lack of physical or mental energy. To be clinically diagnosed with fatigue, you should present with three key components:

- Unable to initiate activities (without medical reason to support why)
- Increase in fatigue, decreased capacity to maintain activities
- Difficulty with concentration, memory, and emotional stability

Fatigue is more than just a lazy person saying, "But I'm too tired to do. . . ." Fatigue is a real condition and very connected to sleep disturbances, affecting 10 to 35 percent of the population. It can result from acute sleep deprivation (less than twenty-four hours) or from cumulative sleep deprivation that happens over several days, weeks, or months.

Fatigue can have an impact on three key areas, creating a significant impact on the ability to function well. It can negatively impact *behavioral factors* and motivation to participate in healthy behaviors such as physical

activity, good nutrition, and prioritizing sleep, which can lead to weight gain and nutritional deficiencies. You may be more willing to engage in unhealthy behaviors such as smoking and changes to your sleep quality and quantity.

Physiological factors such as mood regulation, memory, hormone secretion, nervous system activity, inflammatory pathways, and blood pressure management can become impaired or dysfunctional with ineffective sleep and increased fatigue.

The *psychosocial results* of fatigue are usually most noticeable at work and at home, significantly contributing to decreased stress tolerance, increased conflicts, and difficulty recovering. All of these pathways have been linked either directly or indirectly to sleep disturbances, making them very treatable.

Some people struggle with fatigue more than others. Continue working on sleep hygiene strategies and other behavior modification, as these will help you reduce your fatigue, but you're going to need to pull out some extra tips to feel more alert during the day.

Promoting Wakefulness

Use bright light therapy in the morning within fifteen minutes of waking to reset circadian rhythms (especially in the winter or if you're a shift worker) and to promote wakefulness. This can also be used in the early afternoon when crashing/feeling fatigued, as long as it does not interrupt a normal sleep rhythm.

> *Light therapy can be achieved by either going outside and getting unprotected exposure to the sun or by using a light box. The bright light helps to stimulate chemicals in the brain to set a normal circadian rhythm, giving the cues that it's time to wake up. It usually takes a few weeks of consistent light exposure to become effective. Light therapy can also be used to help reduce the effects of Seasonal Affective Disorder (SAD).*

> **Consult with your physician to determine if using a light box is appropriate for you.*

Schedule physical exercise earlier in the day.

Exercise can be stimulating both physically and mentally. Ensure that you are taking enough downtime between exercise and bedtime so that activity does not interfere with sleep.

Take frequent breaks to move around if sedentary at work or home. Schedule a snack or beverage just prior to the period of fatigue.

This may not be an effective strategy for anyone trying to lose weight! Consider what type of snacks or beverages you are consuming and whether or not the calories are appropriate for your health goals.

Drink a small caffeinated beverage.

Schedule it 30–60 minutes before you need the alert-providing benefits.

If there is no change in fatigue, consider a trial of sleep compression to rule out sleep quality issues—we'll address this in the next section!

Naps

Naps can be used occasionally and are helpful for people who have not yet achieved an optimal sleep schedule, as they can provide several additional hours of alertness. Naps should not be used by anyone who is performing sleep compression therapy, as it tends to reduce the drive to fall asleep and can be counterproductive.

If needed, use a well-timed nap completed prior to 3 p.m. for 15 to 30 minutes and up to 45 minutes. Set an alarm to make sure you actually get up. Your nap must be timed properly to be effective. What does "timed properly" mean? Early enough in the day not to disrupt sleep, or intentionally planned in the late afternoon for night-shift workers who don't sleep well during the day.

Naps can significantly reduce sleepiness and fatigue and improve mood and performance. One of the best strategies to reduce fatigue is to

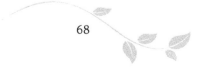

either extend total sleep time or eliminate sleep fragmentation. If you already have broken sleep, extending your sleep duration may lead to more fragmentation, so a planned nap may be a temporary bridge to help you achieve more total sleep time in your day.

Take a "Caffa-Nap"

Need something even better than a nap to get you going? Combine caffeine and naps! It's a great way to supercharge your naps and get even more out of them. Start by grabbing a cup of your favorite caffeinated beverage, then head to a quiet spot for a nap. Ideally, have something like a cup of black coffee, espresso, or strong tea without milk, cream, or sugar in it. The caffeine is what you are going for—not all the added stuff—so leave them out. Set your timer for 30 minutes, then drink your caffeinated beverage as quickly as possible. Don't burn your tongue! Once you've finished your drink of delicious caffeine, snuggle in for a nap until your alarm goes off.

With a *caffa-nap*, you'll wake up refreshed from your nap at the same time the caffeine is starting to hit your system. It works better than using energy drinks because it doesn't have all the sugar and is less impactful on your adrenal glands because you are taking a nap to give your body some extra rest.

Tread lightly and use this with caution! It's not designed to be used over and over again—caffa-naps will definitely create more fatigue if overused. This tip works best if it's only used occasionally, on those days where you just need something to shift you into that next gear for a couple of hours. If you try this more than once in a day, your body is likely going to retaliate and get back at you with some sleepless nights, meaning you'll need caffa-naps even more the next day.

Sleep Compression

Many people have difficulty sleeping, which can be made worse by lying awake in bed for hours on end. By continuing to lie awake in bed, what you are actually doing is creating a negative association with your bed. This is called *stimulus control*.

When you prepare to go to sleep, feelings of fear, frustration, or anxiety are common. They may even be present on a subconscious level without your knowledge. The longer you lie awake in bed, the more you reinforce this association, ultimately making it harder and harder to fall asleep or stay asleep.

Sleep compression is a way of gradually breaking down those negative associations so that you can rebuild a pleasurable association with sleep. This process of re-association is slow and generally hard to change. The longer you have had sleep issues, the longer it will likely take for sleep compression to make an impact on sleep.

In order for changes to occur, patience and consistency are incredibly important. Some people may need up to six months or one year of consistent implementation to rebuild their sleep to an adequate amount.

The purpose of sleep compression is not to get you sleeping as long as possible but to find the optimal balance between sleep quantity and sleep quality. By reducing the amount of time spent in bed (quantity), it may be possible to improve the quality of sleep or total sleep efficiency. Some people may sleep better if they consistently sleep for a shorter time, while other people may need more sleep to feel rested the next day.

Sleep Compression is ideal for people who:
- Consistently have a hard time falling asleep
- Have fragmented sleep and spend more time awake in bed than asleep
- Don't wake up feeling refreshed

Sleep Compression should not be used for anyone who:
- Has bipolar disorder (unless advised to do so by their physician)
- Spends less than five hours in bed/sleeping. These people should consult a sleep specialist to identify other potential health concerns
- Anyone who is operating heavy equipment or vehicles and may be at risk of fatigue-related accidents

Due to a potential reduction in sleep duration, possible adverse effects of sleep compression include:
- A temporary increase in daytime sleepiness/fatigue
- Difficulty concentrating

- Decreased decision-making
- Decreased ability to operate heavy equipment or vehicles

As a result of possible side effects from sleep compression, it is recommended that you be carefully monitored for fatigue and evaluated for safety prior to driving or performing hazardous activities such as working with heavy machinery.

Regardless of how impaired your sleep is, it is important to only restrict your sleep window for an **absolute minimum** of five and a half hours per night, to provide adequate opportunity to get enough sleep. It is likely prudent to advocate for a six hours per night minimum so that you are not cutting into potential sleep time. If you are currently only getting four of sleep hours or less per night, you would still adhere to a minimum window of five and a half hours.

Sleep compression is ideal if you are the kind of person who spends a long time in bed but only gets a few hours of sleep. Take the time you are currently sleeping each night and use that as your starting point; let's say it's six hours, but you're currently in bed for eight hours. Then identify what time you need to get up in the morning. Set your alarm clock for that time and realize that you must get up, even if you don't feel like it. Now, count backward from your wake-up time to determine your sleep time. If you need to be up at 6 a.m., using six hours as your guide, your time to go to sleep would be midnight. Only go to bed when you are drowsy and ready to sleep. Otherwise, you'll be reinforcing the idea of being awake in bed.

If you are the kind of person who usually goes to bed early and reads for a few hours, then you'll be in for a bit of a shock at how late midnight seems as a bedtime. Remember that the point of this is to retrain your body to understand that *your bed equals sleep.* This conditioning helps to strengthen your circadian clock to regulate sleep and wakefulness. The less time you spend in bed doing other things, the stronger this connection gets, which makes it easier to fall asleep and stay asleep over time.

This is where that sleep log can come in handy. While doing sleep compression, track your sleep times every night and pay attention to your sleep efficiency. That's how well you are sleeping. Your goal is to increase your sleep efficiency to over 80 percent *every night*. Once you are hitting that goal, you can add an extra fifteen minutes to your total sleep time, so instead of going to sleep at midnight, now you get to go to sleep at 11:45 p.m.

You can increase your sleep time every week if you are achieving 80 percent efficiency every night. If not, stay put for an extra week—or two or three—until you get there. Turn this into a game to find out where your magic sweet spot is. It's going to be different for everyone. Ideally, over time, you'll find out where you sleep best and wake up feeling refreshed.

If this isn't going well for you, then it may be time to turn to the experts. By working on making positive changes to your sleep, you'll be ahead of the game by the time you get in to see a specialist. They'll appreciate you making an effort to improve your sleep on your own before seeing them.

Shift Work

As you can imagine, pulling together some solid recommendations that apply to every single type of shift work is incredibly challenging. There is little structured literature discussing ideal sleep recommendations for shift workers. This is quite disheartening, since shift workers comprise 17 to 33 percent of the North American workforce. While it is impossible to anticipate every single shift combination, the suggestions I'm about to provide should be easily adaptable to any type of shift pattern.

Keep in mind that you have your own unique set of circumstances. You are not treating your specific shift. Therefore, just because the "recommendations state . . . blah, blah, blah," does not mean that this is the only way to adjust your sleep pattern. Use common sense!

Another key to ensuring optimal sleep quality is to keep a sleep log so that you can evaluate your sleep efficiency. If you are achieving close to 80 or 85 percent efficiency, you are doing well. Your efficiency may not be consistent, however, especially as you move through different shifts. Even if your efficiency is high, due to shift variation, you may still express concerns over being tired. Use the suggestions for fatigue management previously discussed. If you are not able to achieve a desired result, this

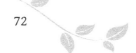

is when you would ask for a referral to a sleep specialist for support in creating a more structured sleep plan.

Tips for All Shift Workers

These suggestions should be implemented in addition to the standard recommendations for sleep hygiene. There are a few points added that are specific to shift workers, which have not been previously discussed.

Avoid alcohol, nicotine and other stimulants prior to bedtime.

Watch diet—reduce hard to digest/large meals before bed.

Exercise regularly—avoid vigorous activity three to six hours before bed.

Reduce or avoid light exposure prior to your sleep period. If possible, keep lights in your work environment dim until your shift has left the building. Use blue blocker or amber sunglasses to on the way home from your shift to help reduce light before bed.

Use bright light therapy after waking up from sleep to provide the body with the correct cues that it's time to wake up. If the waking period is nighttime or is during the winter months, light exposure is helpful because these shift workers can get little to no natural light exposure.

Plan social time with friends and family so that you are not excluded from social relationships.

> *Shift workers often end up isolated due to their unusual shifts, which may lead to depression, anxiety, or other mental health concerns. Maintain social connections, healthy relationships, and support networks.*

Sleep aids (hypnotics/sedatives) are not great for long-term use. Their effectiveness wears off, and the need for a higher dosage increases over time. Instead, use these drugs intermittently or use other sleep strategies to help improve sleep quality, and always as prescribed.

> *Shift workers tend to use sleep aids more, as it can be more challenging to sleep during the day or fall asleep when their bodies think they are in a different time zone. Working with a sleep*

specialist can help to identify what type of sleep aids offer the least side effects with the greatest benefit.

As we age, it becomes harder to switch between shifts due to natural changes in our circadian rhythms. Consider changing to a different shift— or retiring earlier, if at all possible.

Shift work is hard at any age but can become more challenging with age due to natural changes in circadian rhythms. Identify the long-term impact on health, especially in those who have disrupted sleep rhythms, to determine if shift work is still right for you.

Fixed Schedules

Permanent evenings or nights (schedule is classified as shift work due to irregular hours but is always the same hours)

This is the easiest type of shift work to establish or maintain good, high-quality sleep. These workers should keep a regular sleep schedule, even if it is different hours than a typical sleep schedule. For example, a worker who always works nights could set this as their normal routine, and stay on a similar sleep schedule even on days off. They could come home and eat a light meal, have a wind-down period, and then go to sleep for seven to nine hours. If these workers need to adjust their schedules on their days off, they could follow the rotating shift recommendations below.

These schedules are the easiest in which to plan for a sleep routine, as they are much more predictable. Identify a sleep schedule that is realistic for you to have optimal alertness in your job while still allowing time for social connections. Having such a strict sleep schedule that it does not allow for social time isn't healthy either.

Rotating Schedules

Fixed rotating (e.g., "four on, four off" or "one week days, one week nights," always the same predictable pattern)

With fixed, rotating shifts, workers are able to anticipate shifts ahead of time and can create a sleep plan for each night of their rotation. For

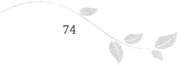

example, day one of the rotation would always be the same routine; day two might be different from day one but is always the same, etc. These shift workers should look ahead to the next day and plan their sleep routine for their next shift.

Random rotating (e.g., "four on, five off," "four on, seven off," or a "days/evenings/nights line")

These types of rotations are always changing or have a long, predictable pattern, where the schedule repeats every ten weeks, etc. These workers have the hardest time creating good sleep patterns, as there is literally no consistency in sleep. Having solid sleep hygiene practices is vital for these shift workers.

On-Call

These workers have incredible variation in their shifts and have to sleep with "one eye open" because they could get called in at any moment. Follow sleep recommendations for the type of shift being worked and consider using naps to make up for the lack of quality sleep.

Rotating schedules tend to be more challenging in terms of providing general suggestions, as there are several types of rotating schedules. Here are a few options of transitions to different shifts:

Day to Day

Go to sleep at the same time and wake up at the same time, allowing for seven to nine hours of consolidated sleep.

Day to Night

Delay your sleep schedule by a few hours on the last day or two prior to the shift change to transition to nights easier. A longer nap (60–90 minutes) in the afternoon of the first night shift, followed by bright light therapy, can help to make the night shift go by easier.

Night to Day

After the last night shift, follow suggestions from the fixed schedule, but instead of sleeping for seven to nine hours, set an alarm to allow for a few hours of sleep. Then get up at midday, get bright light exposure, and perform low-level activity (e.g., grocery shopping, going for a walk) and plan to go to bed at the same time you would for a day shift. An alarm will likely be needed to wake up the next morning at the normal time for a day shift.

Night to Night

This is similar to the day to day shift transition, just on opposite hours. Go to sleep at the same time and wake up at the same time, allowing for seven to nine hours of consolidated sleep.

Evening Shifts

These shifts are the in-between world of shifts, and times can vary dramatically on when these shifts start and end. Again, the goal is to get seven to nine hours of sleep each night—the actual time to go to bed and get up are adjusted to suit the shift.

> *Random rotating schedules are the hardest to plan for a sleep routine, as they are much less predictable. Identify a long-term sleep schedule so that you can learn how to adjust your sleep to match the work schedule. Follow the same suggestions as a fixed schedule.*

For the general shift suggestions (day to day, night to day, etc.), use common sense first. You'll also want to consider other needs such as childcare, social commitments, etc. The suggestions are to help create an ideal sleep pattern, which in some cases is not possible. Sometimes, a compromise needs to be made. However, recognize that this may have positive or negative implications in other aspects of your overall well-being. Try to reduce the stress around this decision and recognize that you can't control every aspect of your life.

Pillar 2: Nutrition

"Let food be thy medicine and medicine be thy food."

—HIPPOCRATES

"The eighteenth century was the century of political rights; the nineteenth century was the century of women's rights; the twentieth century was the century of civil rights. The challenge of the twenty-first century will be the struggle for food and farming rights."

—SALLY FALLON,
PRESIDENT OF THE WESTON A. PRICE FOUNDATION

Chapter Five

Nutrition Essentials

*I*f your goal is to be as optimally healthy as you can, one of the best places to start is with your nutrition. Keep in mind that a lot of the nutrition recommendations out there are based on making sure that people have **sufficient** nutrients, not **optimal** nutrients. The recommended daily intake (RDI) does not focus on providing optimal nutrition, nor does it focus on how to improve someone's current state of health. To aim for optimal health, you will need to look at how you interpret standard nutrition recommendations.

To start with, let's look at what optimal nutrition is and what the goals of optimal nutrition should be. Here are a few definitions of optimal nutrition:

- "A functional marker reaches an 'optimal value' or plateau, beyond which it is no longer affected by intake stores of the nutrient." —The National Institutes of Health
- "A diet conducive to the most favorable activity or function." —Irwin H. Rosenberg, *Journal of Nutrition*
- "Giving yourself the best possible intake of nutrients to allow your body to be as healthy and to work as well as it possibly can. It is not a set of rules." —Institute for Optimum Nutrition

Given those definitions, I'd say that our traditional nutrition recommendations are far from meeting the ability to create optimal nutrition. We've got a long road ahead of us to formally change nutrition recommendations. However, you can start today by learning how to start eating for optimal health.

Before we delve too far down the nutrition rabbit hole, let's start with reviewing the fundamentals of nutrition that are important. I'm always surprised by the number of people who have never been taught the difference between nutrients and food groups. I feel it's important to go back to the basics.

Nutrients include protein, carbohydrates, fat, vitamins, minerals, and water. A food is inherently made up some combination of nutrients to provide our bodies with energy to survive and hopefully thrive. It's important to distinguish between food groups and nutrients because **your body does not need to eat specific food groups**.

We've been indoctrinated to think that we need dairy products and grain products to survive, and that's simply not true. While your body needs proteins, carbohydrates, and fats, there's absolutely no daily requirement for any specific food groups to be consumed. Dairy and grains aren't all bad. They may be beneficial for some people. However, they should be evaluated on a case-by-case basis rather than recommended as a blanket policy for everyone to consume.

Proteins

Proteins are broken down into amino acids, some of which are essential because our bodies do not produce them. What that means is that we need to consume foods rich in the amino acids we are lacking in order to meet our bodies' needs. The role of protein is to build and repair tissues (e.g., bone, muscle, skin), synthesize and regulate other molecules (enzymes and hormones), and form antibodies. If you like statistics, each gram of protein has four calories.

Real-food sources of protein come from meat or fish of any kind and are considered to be **complete proteins** because they contain all of the

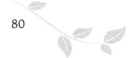

amino acids in order to be broken down in the body. **Incomplete proteins** lack certain amino acids and cannot be fully processed unless they are combined with the remainder of amino acids. Examples of incomplete proteins are beans and legumes that would need to be paired with a food like rice to complete their amino acid profile.

It's also important to note that all protein formation stops when amino acids are missing, which prevents cells from becoming imbalanced. (Let's face it—who wants half a muscle cell floating around? Who knows what harm that would do! Fortunately, that can't happen.) Balancing amino acids is especially important if you are vegetarian or vegan, as you may not be getting a proper balance of amino acids. The body has poor storage of amino acids and needs daily sources to maintain adequate levels of protein.

You'll likely want to consider higher protein requirements if you need to lose weight. That's because of the benefits protein provides for building and repairing tissues such as muscle mass. This will help you maintain or increase muscle mass and positively impact your metabolism. You'll also want to consider whether the foods you are eating have other nutrients combined in them. Foods such as quinoa, nuts, and beans all have protein but are also rich in carbohydrates, which will need to be taken into account, especially since statistically, approximately 40 to 50 percent of people are overweight or obese.

For an average person (80 kg or 180 lbs) who wants to lose weight, your protein requirements are around 120 grams of protein each day (at a rate of 1.5 grams of protein per kilogram of body weight). That works out to three meals of 30 grams of protein and two snacks of 12 grams of protein.

Here are some examples of how much food you need to eat just to get 12 grams of protein, which is a common serving size for most snacks:

	Serving Size	Amount of Carbohydrates
Salmon	54 g	0 g
Eggs	2 eggs	0 g
Beef	1.3 oz	0 g
Almonds	46 almonds	10 g

	Serving Size	Amount of Carbohydrates
Peanut butter	2 tbsp	16 g
Broccoli	2 cups	20 g
Lentils	3/4 cup	26 g
Lima beans	1 cup	36 g
Quinoa	3 cups	76 g

The crazy part is when you look at how many carbohydrates you are getting with each serving of protein. One serving of carbohydrates is only 15 grams. In this small sample of foods, you'll note that some foods like quinoa have up to five servings of carbohydrates just to get 12 grams of protein. I have nothing against quinoa, and actually quite like it, but I really struggle when my clients eat quinoa as their sole protein source because they argue that it is *technically* a whole protein source.

Compare this to meat sources of protein, and there's no competition. Most people eat far too many carbohydrates anyway, so unless you are vegetarian or vegan, it would make more sense to eat whole-protein sources instead of alternative protein options. A reasonable amount of protein for most people to aim for is 1.5 grams of protein per kilogram of body weight, as long as you don't have early-stage kidney issues.

Carbohydrates

Carbohydrates are broken down into sugar molecules to provide energy for the body and are termed according to the complexity of the sugar molecule. A single sugar is called a **monosaccharide** (glucose, fructose), two sugars are called **disaccharides** (sucrose—made up of glucose and fructose), and more than two are termed **oligosaccharides** (yes, another big word that I won't talk about again). These three types of sugars are commonly referred to as simple sugars. Some examples of simple sugars are honey and fruit. **Polysaccharides** or complex sugars are starches such as potatoes, rice, wheat, glycogen (glycerol and fatty acid), and cellulose or fiber.

Your next question should be, "What is the function of carbohydrates in the body?" They have lots of important roles, like breaking down into sugar molecules for energy (remember this point for later—you will be tested on this!). They also support immune function, fuel tissue regrowth/joint fluidity, and are involved in cell recognition, nerve/muscle function, and metabolism regulation.

Due to their numerous functions, carbohydrates are an important part of a healthy diet. That being said, it is important to remember that there are *no essential* carbohydrates.

That's right: There's absolutely no daily minimum requirement for carbohydrates. Without adequate carbohydrate, the body is able to pull energy from the other nutrients to perform the same functions. It wouldn't be wise to pull all carbohydrates from your diet because of the benefits you get from them, but perhaps we should reconsider the common daily recommendations.

Our bodies do need a small amount of carbohydrates for essential brain function, but only about 30 grams a day for a very low-carb ketogenic diet. This energy can come from lower-carbohydrate foods such as vegetables. Low-carbohydrate diets typically limit consumption to around 8 percent of total daily calories from carbohydrates. This varies greatly from most recommendations, which suggest that between 40 and 60 percent of all calories come from carbohydrates. Based on a 2,000-calorie diet, the Canadian Diabetes Association recommends 130 grams of carbohydrates each day, which is less than 30 percent of carbohydrate calories.

Our bodies do need some carbohydrates to perform all the magic processes we've already talked about, but in my humble opinion, carbohydrate recommendations are much higher than what is needed for optimal nutrition. I personally would like to see carbohydrate recommendations changed so that they are based on activity level and body composition.

New recommendations should also focus on eating unrefined carbohydrate sources that tend to be higher in fiber and lower in glycemic (sugar) value. A person who is sedentary or overweight (most of us) needs significantly fewer carbohydrates than someone who is lean or training for an endurance event like an Ironman triathlon or a marathon. I suspect that this recommendation hasn't been made because it's not a one-size-fits-all approach, and would be more difficult for people to understand. Until we reach that point, a realistic carbohydrate recommendation would be around 100 grams of carbohydrates per day or potentially even less for those who are sedentary or need to lose weight.

Fat

Despite popular belief, fat does not make you fat. People become fat from an excess of calories compared to their energy expenditure, or because of hormonal imbalances.

Now that we've dispelled that myth, let's look at fat as a nutrient. Sitting at a whopping nine calories per gram, fat is vital to creating optimal health. Fat is used as a storage for energy (which is why it has nine calories instead of four per gram). It also transfers fat-soluble nutrients (D, E, K, and A vitamins), provides satiation (that feeling of being full), builds cellular membranes, repairs damage from chemicals, and provides insulation to the body. Fat is used to build hormones (like cortisol and testosterone), plus the lining of the nervous system, and it is involved in liver, blood, and skin health. Protein and fat can also slow the absorption of carbohydrates, and fats turn into lipids when they are broken down.

Similar to carbohydrates, fats are named according to their chemical structure (snore!) based on their carbon chains. **Triglycerides** are some of the most common types of fats, which are three fatty acids on a glycerol backbone. **Saturated fats** are carbon and fatty acids linked by a single bond and have hydrogen atoms attached to every available bonding site. Saturated fats are solid at room temperature and are commonly found in animal fats like lard, butter, margarine, and palm/coconut oils. Saturated fats are recommended to make up less than 7 to 10 percent of daily caloric intake and have historically been blamed for many health issues. New research suggests that saturated fats may not be as bad as we once thought, and that they are likely fairly benign in a diet lower in carbohydrates. Their risk of causing cardiovascular disease is ultimately unknown at this point.

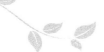

Unsaturated fats are linked by one or more double bonds and do not have hydrogen atoms at every available bonding site. These fats are liquid at room temperature and tend to come from plant oils (avocado, olive, flax) and fish oils EPA and DHA. To break down unsaturated fats even more, **monounsaturated fats** have one carbon-to-carbon bond that is not saturated by hydrogen, like oleic acid (found in olive oil, canola oil, and avocados). **Polyunsaturated fats** have two or more carbon-to-carbon bonds not saturated by hydrogen.

Essential fats, those fats that we must consume from our diet in order to be healthy, are omega-3 and omega-6. Currently, most people have an average omega-3/omega-6 ratio of one to twenty, when we ideally want that ratio to be closer to one to two for optimal health.

The omega-3s that we are all significantly lacking include alpha-linolenic acid, EPA, and DHA, which come from flaxseed, pumpkin, hemp seed, walnut, fish oil, and grass-fed/finished beef. The omega-6s are linoleic acid, gamma-linolenic acid, and arachidonic acid, which come from foods like grapeseed oil, sesame oil, safflower oil, sunflower oil, borage oil, evening primrose oil, beef fat, and egg yolk.

Have I lost you yet? I'm not even sure *I* fully understand what all that means. Oy vey!

Additionally, I should mention that while there's a lot of talk about how horrible cholesterol is, and how important it is to cut all cholesterol out of your diet, it simply *isn't the case*. **Cholesterol** is a fat-soluble liquid from animal products that forms hormones and cell membranes in the brain and nerves. It's also naturally produced in the body. I don't know about you, but I think it's a really good idea to keep those nerve cell membranes intact and help our brains work as best as they can. I'm not saying we should eat cholesterol-rich foods with reckless abandon, but we do want to make sure that we are eating (or naturally producing) enough to keep our brains and nerves healthy.

What is becoming clear in terms of fat is that the **quality** of fat is much more important than the **quantity**. Trans-fats should be eliminated because of their harmful effects. Higher omega-3 diets can decrease cardiovascular risk, and reduce components of cholesterol including triglycerides, small dense LDL and LDL-C. High-fat diets may cause an increased cancer risk, although that risk may be mitigated if better-quality fat is consumed—only further research will tell! It seems reasonable to consume around 20 to 35 percent of your total calories from good-quality fats, with 10 percent of that total coming from omega-3 fats.

Vitamins

Vitamins are organic compounds (containing carbon) that are found in plants and animals in nature. They are critical for helping with the many enzyme processes that occur in the body. There are twenty-one vitamins, with five being fat-soluble and the other sixteen being water-soluble. (New research, however, suggests a twenty-second essential vitamin: the fatty acids that we discussed in the previous section.) I won't bore you with all the details of every vitamin, its purpose, and recommended dose—at this point, you just need to know that we need *all* of them!

Vitamins affect coenzymes and help convert protein, carbohydrates, and fat into usable energy sources. Vitamins form components of body tissues such as the calcium in bone or the amino acids in muscle. They help with cellular reactions, metabolism, digestion, and disease resistance, and they are prohormones and antioxidants.

Deficiencies of vitamins can create behavioral issues or mood disturbances. Health care practitioners, unfortunately, typically treat mental health with medication first, rather than going back to the basics and ensuring that the patient is getting adequate vitamin intake. By improving your diet, you can likely eliminate or at least decrease many symptoms of anxiety, depression, and irritability, without the nasty side effects that drugs carry.

Minerals

Minerals are made up of elements, the building blocks of matter, including carbon, hydrogen, oxygen, and nitrogen. They get broken down into

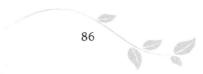

ash, inorganic substance in the soil. There are twenty-six minerals, with eleven macrominerals (big), and fifteen microminerals (small). The body can't manufacture minerals, so they must be consumed in the diet. They are considered essential when deficiency symptoms present and then go away with an intake of the same mineral. Minerals help with the body's acid/base balance, fluid balance, hormone production, and metabolism. Minerals also help with heart/muscle function and nerve conductivity, and are present in protein, enzymes, blood, and some vitamins.

Since society has turned to large-scale farming practices with mono-crops (restricting one type of vegetable per field), our soil quality has dramatically plummeted, leaving our crops with few vitamins and minerals. Remember that we need the vitamins and minerals to get the health benefits of the food, so we are essentially growing tasteless food lacking in nutrition. What's the point?

To combat this, many people turn to supplements, which, in some ways, may not be any better. The supplement industry is poorly regulated, and there are thousands of poor-quality supplements on the market that provide little benefit. We urgently need to shift our farming practices to replace the vitamins and minerals we are so badly lacking.

Water

Around 60 to 75 percent of the body is made up of water, and we can survive only a few days without water. It is used for temperature regulation, transporting nutrients, and electrolytes. Water helps with chemical reactions and energy formation and detoxifies the body by removing waste.

There is a delicate balance between dehydration and water intoxication, and the body displays harsh effects if this balance goes too far in either direction. When looking at optimal water intake, there are several factors to consider. Obligatory water losses are daily water losses that we can't consciously change or control, such as urine production, breathing, and normal daily sweat. Other factors that help us determine an appropriate rate for hydration are gender, age, the size of the person, the type of diet, their environment (altitude and temperature), activity level, and sweat rate.

The lowest daily recommendation I've seen was 455 milliliters per day, and the highest was 16 liters per day. That's a huge range and will require some discretion before deciding how much to drink. What seems to be common and reasonable is to consume 1 milliliter of water for every calorie you consume. For someone eating a 2,000-calorie diet, you would want to consume 2,000 milliliters (2 liters) of water each day. If you live in a hot climate or are very active, it would be wise to increase this recommendation and decrease it if you have kidney failure or congestive heart failure.

Summary

Think of your diet as a pyramid. Start with a solid foundation—as wide of a base of support as possible. Often times, I see clients come in with really detailed questions about the latest media trend, but they don't even know what a carbohydrate food is. There's absolutely no point in chipping away at the top of the pyramid when the bottom is crumbling. Eventually, it will come tumbling down. Go back to the basics before you start working on the larger details.

Let's review what these nutrients do:

Proteins
- 4 calories per gram
- *Function*: build and repair tissues, synthesize and regulate other molecules (enzymes and hormones), form antibodies
- Balance amino acids and consume complete protein sources

Carbohydrates
- 4 calories per gram
- *Function*: energy, immune function, tissue regrowth/joint fluidity, cell recognition, nerve/muscle function, and metabolism regulation
- Ideally, eat unrefined, unprocessed, high-fiber, low-sugar sources

Fats
- 9 calories per gram
- *Function*: build hormones/lining of the nervous system, involved in liver/blood and skin health
- Slow the absorption of carbohydrates
- Quality over quantity

Vitamins
- *Function*: convert protein, carbs, and fat into usable energy sources, help coenzymes, form components of body tissues, help with cellular reactions, metabolism, digestion, disease resistance, pro-hormones, antioxidants, balance mood/behaviors

Minerals
- *Function*: acid/base balance, fluid balance, hormone production and metabolism, heart/muscle function, nerve conductivity, present in protein, enzymes, blood, and some vitamins

Water
- *Function*: temperature regulation, transport nutrients/electrolytes, chemical reactions, energy formation, detoxification by removing waste
- Consider water losses when deciding on optimal water intake

Chapter Six

What Should You Eat?

I've come across many people who swear that they eat right and even brag to me about how healthy they are eating. This is a red flag in my book, and it often reveals that you aren't eating as well as you think you are.

It is a *huge* lie to claim that there is "one master diet" that will work for everyone. Our nutritional requirements vary exceedingly depending on our health, activity levels, stress levels, the environment in which we live, and so many other factors. This is why there are thousands of fad diets that claim to be successful, because even as absurd as some of them are, some people will try them and successfully lose weight.

Through a large analysis of journal articles and recommendations from numerous health organizations (Canada's Food Guide, USDA Portion Plate, Diabetes Associations, etc.) as well as comparing several different diets (e.g., vegan, vegetarian, paleo, Zone, DASH, raw food, etc.), I have been able to identify some key components of nutrition that are consistent across all of the different fad diets.

As I mentioned, there is no one diet that is perfect for everyone, so you may need to play around a bit to find what works best for you. Knowledge of nutrition is also increasing at light speed, to the point that health recommendations can't keep up. Unless you are actively learning new material from credible sources, your nutrition knowledge is probably already out of date.

In this section, you're not going to get specific recommendations on RDIs, percentages of macro or micronutrients, or a specific meal plan, because that style of nutrition teaching simply doesn't work. If that were the extent of my recommendations, you wouldn't learn anything in the long run. You would simply become dependent on each new plan coming out and telling you what to eat. What I will give you are some general guidelines for deciding on whether a diet is healthy for you, and to identify if the diet will help you achieve optimal health.

The essential components that a healthy diet must include are:

- Food security
- Affordable
- Low in processed foods
- High in nutrients
- Variety
- Long-term sustainability
- Hydration
- Fuel for activity level
- Social component
- Balancing blood sugars

Food Security

The pillars of health are those key components that need to be in place in order to be able to achieve health. Not even optimal health—just health. When we look at nutrition, our pillars of health really come down to being able to have food security. Regardless of what your goals are, if you can't afford to eat, you won't have the options to make better choices. You need to address food security first before you can start trying to follow specific recommendations to eat organic produce or consume a certain ratio of nutrients. You want to start with the basics and be able to afford food first.

If you aren't able to meet your basic needs or are struggling to eat healthier foods, that's when you can look into food subsidy programs. Most cities have a food bank, which is a good start for getting back on your feet; however, they often have limited choices and poor quality of foods available. Some cities also have a Good Food Box program, which is a subsidized fruit and vegetable program that skips the markup of grocery stores and commonly sells boxes for around one to two dollars per pound instead of the two to three dollars it would be in a grocery store.

Another way to provide food security for yourself and others is to take advantage of a lunch program at your workplace or school. I remember, from a previous job, that for some children, the school lunch program provided the only meal that child might get that day. It's pretty sad that in westernized cultures we still have people who can't afford to buy basic foods. We need to provide our children with healthy foods so that their brains can develop properly and they can grow into healthy adults. As for adults, they need to get enough nutrition to perform and excel in their jobs and lives.

Another thing you can do to create a more stable food system is to start growing your own vegetables or fruit. There are hundreds of resources on the internet on how to build a tiny garden by using a fence as a vertical frame for your vegetables or using planters or pots. Front lawns are typically a decent size and can easily be turned into a combination of a vegetable and flower garden to keep it looking nice all year. If you don't have a yard, start up a community garden plot with your community association. There are also lots of resources available online on what types of plants grow best in your climate zone, along with tips on what plants to put near each other to help naturally deter pests and attract bees. The plants that I can grow in my home in Calgary are going to be much different than what you could grow in San Francisco, London, or Adelaide. Growing seasons also vary dramatically. For about half the year, it's simply too cold for me to grow anything outside, which makes it that much more special when I can work in my garden.

The basics of growing a garden are all the same, regardless of where you grow. You need four key components to grow healthy food: healthy soil, good-quality seeds, water, and sunshine. That's it! Now, the specifics get a bit more complicated depending on your region, growing season, types of plants, but you don't need a PhD in botany to grow a garden! It really doesn't take an expert to grow a bit of lettuce. Growing even a small amount of vegetables will relieve some of the burden from your food system and will make a big difference when combined with the efforts of others.

If you are in a position to be able to afford better-quality food, buy organic, pastured, or grass-fed meats and sustainably raised foods. By doing this, you are showing our food producers that there is a need and demand for better-quality products. The more that we as consumers demand that better-quality foods be produced, the more production will increase, and the cost will come down due to increased efficiency.

It's also important to realize that there is a spectrum of food quality. Don't avoid all produce just because you can't afford to eat organic foods. You'll be missing out on valuable nutrients that are important for achieving optimal nutrition. There's no solid evidence supporting that organic fruits and vegetables are more nutritious. However, you may reduce your exposure to pesticides by eating organic.

Affordable

Eat the highest-quality food that you can afford without breaking the bank. Americans spend only 6 percent of their total income on food. Canadians are marginally better at 9 percent, while other westernized countries spend a significantly higher proportion (10 to 12 percent) of their total income on food. By putting a higher proportion of income into better-quality food, you are investing in your health and will reduce the amount of money needed to treat chronic conditions down the line.

You can also eat wholesome foods at an affordable price by investing more of your time in food preparation. By buying in bulk, produce is much more affordable than purchasing individually packaged items. You will need to develop basic cooking skills such as chopping or peeling vegetables, but the gains in health will be unmatched.

Low in Processed Foods

We know from thousands of highly researched journal articles that processed foods are connected to cancer risk, diabetes, cholesterol, weight gain, and so many other negative health effects. You'll want to really learn what it means to eat processed foods, as many people may not fully understand.

There is a huge misconception of what "processed" really means and how it differs from *real* food. A patient of mine, Sherry, told me, "I don't eat very many processed foods. I never eat fast food, and I'm having a lot of fruit smoothies." After completing an evaluation of her diet, I discovered that she was consuming lots of juice, pasta, bread, cereals, crackers, and deli meats, which are all processed. Sherry thought that processed foods were only pre-packaged meals like lasagna, microwave dinners, or pre-made pizza.

Just because something can go in your mouth or into your digestive tract does not mean that the item can be classified as "food." A whole food is an item that can be found outside of human influence such as an apple, a cashew, a coconut, beef, fish, or wild rice. Food, ideally, is anything that comes naturally from the earth that is not altered, modified, or processed. Food can be raised or grown, like animals or vegetables, and is alive prior to consumption.

By contrast, processed food or a food product is a combination of foods and/or chemicals that have been subjected to some type of processing to make them more palatable or accessible to eat. Since there is a wide range of processing, not every processed food should be looked at as bad or the root of all evil. For example, cut broccoli sold in a package is technically processed, but broccoli is commonly identified as a health food. (Generally, most processed food isn't going to help you create optimal health.)

Overall, we live in a busy, fast-paced society, and convenience is supremely important to most people. Consider other situations and events that may increase your need for processed foods. If you were going to go on a back-country backpacking trip for a week and needed to carry all of your food with no ability to replenish your supplies other than water, you would be reliant on freeze-dried or dehydrated foods. It would be extremely challenging to pack a week's worth of fresh food without risking food poisoning. That doesn't even account for the *weight* of the foods or the amount of space that that much fresh food would take up. The key is to eat real, whole food as often as possible.

Here are some telltale signs of processed food:

- It has a label with two or more ingredients
- The label makes a health claim (e.g., high fiber, low sodium, high antioxidants)
- It has a logo from an association (e.g., Diabetes Association/Heart & Stroke)
- It has a recognizable slogan or jingle

When was the last time you saw an ad campaign for spinach? Let's say that the spinach producers of the world got together and pooled all their marketing dollars to launch a massive campaign. They put out billboards and took out Facebook ads to attract more customers and promote the health of spinach. This ad campaign could talk about the fiber content of spinach or how the amount of iron in it makes it a super food. Do you think spinach sales would go up if that happened? Absolutely. There have been instances of vegetable producers joining together to make a point, such as in 1990, when truckloads of broccoli showed up at the White House after President H. W. Bush remarked that he didn't like broccoli. But typically, producers of real food don't take out those types of ads because they don't need to make those types of claims. Most people *know* that spinach is healthy. Not everyone likes spinach, but overall, we know that it's a health food.

The foods that *need* to make claims are doing so simply to sell you a product and stand out from their competition. These foods are *food products* that are produced to be sold to you. They aren't generally designed with your optimal health in mind; most are designed to increase sales within a company.

Shopping for food is no different than shopping for cars. One is more fuel efficient, one has a better safety rating, and one is much more stylish. It's up to you as the consumer to decide if you want to buy the Cadillac

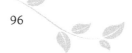

of foods (like broccoli) or the lemon. (Get it? A lemon of a car, not the produce. . . ? Okay, maybe not so funny.)

By shifting your focus away from processed foods—especially carbohydrates that are processed and refined—you will have an easier time losing weight, balancing your blood sugars, and decreasing inflammation in your body. Choose carbohydrates that have a lower glycemic index and higher fiber content (think berries instead of a banana) as well as being whole or unrefined, such as wild rice instead of rice pasta.

High in Nutrients

Move away from the "food group" philosophy and toward a *nutrient* philosophy. Eat nutrients: proteins, carbohydrates, fats, vitamins, minerals, and water. You do not specifically need to consume milk and milk alternatives, meat and meat alternatives, and grain products, as the current system is telling you. Choose foods that are naturally high in vitamins and minerals. Foods are the most nutrient-dense when they are fresh, so choose fresh as often as possible.

Variety

You want to eat a wide variety of foods. Most people tend to get little variety, consuming the same types of foods all year.

To have variety in your diet, you don't need to spend a ton of money buying foods shipped from all over the world. In each climate zone, you are typically able to grow many more varieties of vegetables and fruits than you might see in a grocery store. Look at heirloom tomatoes—there are several different varietals that never make it to the grocery store because they may not look or smell a certain way. As a result, these heirloom varieties of foods are typically not even available for us to eat.

Imagine if you expanded the variety of the common vegetables that you eat. Instead of just eating carrots, peas, and beans, by having different types of each, you would significantly expand the variety of nutrients that you are exposed to. If you like carrots, try purple carrots, yellow carrots, orange carrots. If you like beans, try pole beans, purple beans, blue beans, green beans. . . . Get the picture?

Long-Term Sustainability

We need our food system to be sustainable for years to come. At the rate we are consuming food products, we are heavily depleting our soils, resulting in whole foods that lack taste, nutrients, and minerals. Moving forward, our focus on nutrition *has to be* turning our attention to taking care of our soil. We need to replace the nutrients in our soils that have been lacking for years.

It's likely going to take several years of hard work for our soils to recover and become nutrient-rich again, but it will be worth it. As our soil quality gradually improves, the delicious taste and nutrient density of vegetables will return, and health will start to improve as a result. The initial input of replacing those nutrients and minerals in our soil through compost, rotational grazing, rotational crop planting, and companion planting to deter pests will be well worth the effort.

By no means am I claiming to be a farmer or an expert in agriculture. However, I believe that a combined approach to agriculture, using sustainable livestock and plan management systems and new technology, will improve our food quality while maintaining higher production levels.

Hydration

You want to make sure that you aren't overhydrating or underhydrating. When James came to see me, he was drinking ten liters of water each day and was barely sleeping because he was waking up every hour to pee. He complained of excessive thirst and was unable to satiate it regardless of how much he drank. With his blood sugars well managed, I knew it wasn't diabetes causing his thirst, but rather, his body trying to tell him that he needed more sodium. After cutting back James's water intake to four liters each day, he was able to regulate his thirst and return to sleeping through the night.

On the opposite end of the spectrum, Insha was sedentary and did not drink any water because she hated the taste of it. She often had tea with caffeine, and she never felt thirsty. By increasing Insha's intake of herbal tea to 1.5 liters each day, she felt more energetic and noticed that the acne on her face decreased significantly.

The reason you want to have optimal hydration is to flush out the toxins in your body, to help keep your cells working as effectively and efficiently as possible, and to regulate temperature. An easy assessment for hydration is to look at the color of your urine. You want to have relatively clear urine—not necessarily colorless but not the color of tea or cola either. If you take vitamins or eat richly colored vegetables, the color of your urine may be stained yellow or pink, so be aware of these changes.

Fuel for Activity Level

Most people rate their current activity as "moderately active" when, more realistically, they actually fall in the "sedentary" category.

In general, we notoriously overestimate our calorie expenditures and underestimate our calorie consumption. This poor combination leads to weight gain over the years! You'll want to gauge your activity level and plan calorie consumption based on the amount of energy you are burning. If you are gaining unwanted weight or not losing weight while trying to, you are likely consuming too many calories. On the other end, if you are starting to lose weight when you aren't trying to, your calorie intake is too low.

Food is Tied to Social Connections

Lack of social connection is a greater predictor of illness than any specific food choice on its own. When people go on super-strict diets or follow quirky health trends that leave them with only a few food options, their social connections suffer.

I was struggling with some gastrointestinal issues for years and couldn't find the source of my issues. I started on an elimination diet to pull out the most common allergens that might be upsetting my belly. I did that diet faithfully for months with no success, so my diet was reduced again to find the culprit.

This continued for almost a year, and by that time, I was only eating a few foods with no change to my symptoms and had absolutely no social life. I became lonely and isolated, frequently feeling depressed. I had lost all hope that I'd ever be able to eat normal food again and missed hanging out with my friends. I joked that I should go on a "Twinkies and tequila" diet. Since nothing else seemed to work, I thought I might as well enjoy myself.

It was when I started to work with a naturopath that I started to understand how much of a difference social connection can make to a person's health—much more so than following a specific diet. He even said that patients who occasionally have beer and pizza and have a lot of fun doing it *can* be healthier than isolated people on super-clean, healthy diets.

Not that I'm advocating for a beer and pizza or Twinkies and tequila diet, but you need to learn how to have fun while making responsible food choices that are in line with your health goals. It's common to feel that since you can't eat certain foods, you can't be social because so many social engagements revolve around food. I learned to eat most of my meal at home before going out to social events, but I still snacked on safe foods while I was out so I could reconnect with my social networks. By spending more time having fun and being social, I was spending less time focusing on "poor me," which made a significant improvement in my health and mood. I've found the same results working with many of my clients.

Balancing Blood Sugars

You'll want to balance your insulin and blood sugar because of the connection to other hormones in the body. Even if blood sugar lab results look normal, unless you are tracking your blood sugar several times a day, you truly have no idea how you are processing sugars. This type of tracking also doesn't account for your insulin release to control the number of carbohydrates you are consuming.

The way our current health care system is set up is that blood sugars only get flagged once they hit a pre-diabetic or diabetic range. Once you've been diagnosed with type two diabetes, you have already lost about 40 percent to 50 percent of the function of the cells in your pancreas. It

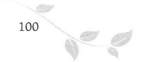

seems really silly to me that we let people lose at least 40 percent function before we even do anything about it. This is what is currently happening.

As someone who wants to be proactive with their health, make sure that you are doing the right things with nutrition to control your blood sugar. You'll also want to investigate other areas of your life that have an impact on blood sugar such as sleep, stress level, infections, or medications that may cause a blood sugar increase. You'll want to tighten up the carbohydrate recommendations if you have difficulty processing sugar, are insulin resistant, need to lose weight, or are trying to reduce inflammation in your body.

At the beginning of this chapter, I mentioned that people who brag about how healthy they eat usually aren't doing as well as they think. An example of this is evident in the many people who eat oatmeal for breakfast. Marketing has told you that oatmeal is a healthy, balanced breakfast and high in fiber. In theory, this is correct, but most of my clients are eating instant oatmeal. You just rip the package open and add hot water. This type of oatmeal isn't much different than eating white bread or pure sugar for breakfast. Instant oatmeal breaks down very quickly due to its lack of fiber, resulting in a rapid increase in blood sugars, sending you on a sugar roller coaster for the rest of the day.

Many people also think that just by having a small handful of nuts or a bit of peanut butter on their toast, they are balancing their blood sugars. But when you examine the carbohydrates and protein in this option gram for gram, the amount of protein needed in peanut butter to balance the number of carbohydrates in bread becomes unsustainable. It works out to almost four tablespoons of peanut butter to get enough protein to balance the amount of sugar in one slice of bread. However, that peanut butter is also adding more carbohydrates into the equation, creating an even bigger imbalance. We also haven't even considered the fact that those four tablespoons of peanut butter pack around 400 calories into your breakfast, likely adding a dramatic increase of calories into your diet. Most people aren't eating anywhere close to four tablespoons of peanut butter on one piece of bread and likely couldn't do this on a consistent basis without gaining a significant amount of weight.

Blood Sugar Explained

Most people start their day with a cup of coffee or tea and then eat carbohydrate-rich foods. Both of these habits can cause an increase in blood sugar. When blood sugar rises quickly, it also tends to fall quickly. This starts a cascade of hormones in the body, resulting in volatile blood sugar that goes up and down quickly throughout the day. Eating a balanced lunch or dinner does not necessarily reset those hormones. This volatile blood sugar pattern causes periods of fatigue or cravings for sugary or carbohydrate-rich foods, usually in the afternoon or evening.

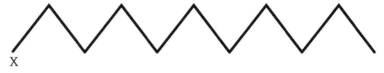

(Imbalanced blood sugar = bad)

After looking at hundreds of diets, one of the most common breakfasts that I see is yogurt, fruit, and berries. Despite being *healthy*, this is not *balanced.* Those foods *all* break down into carbohydrates and drive blood sugars up first thing in the morning. Add a cup of coffee to that picture, and it continues to drive blood sugar imbalances. The result is a mid-morning crash where you need another cup of coffee or a snack to keep going.

Other common times for sugar crashes include that dip just after lunch or mid-afternoon. People often get home from work and are "hangry," that awful hungry-angry feeling where you have no control over what goes into your mouth because you must eat, now! The other most common time I see people having blood sugar issues occurs in those who crave snacks after dinner or for dessert. It's nearly impossible to "out-willpower" yourself when these blood sugar signals are yelling, "feed me sugar." These cravings are all caused by what you ate for breakfast, and they are relatively easy to control once you know what to do.

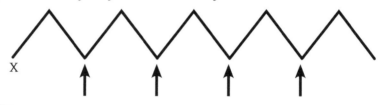

Rather than me telling you to stop having an afternoon or evening snack—which is only patching or covering the symptoms—you should start at the source of the problem and balance your blood sugar from the very beginning of the day. Start the day with an equal amount of protein and carbohydrates, or consume foods that have fewer carbohydrates (e.g., protein and vegetables). Do this gram for gram, not size-based, as different foods come in different serving sizes. This approach to eating will help to level blood sugars, resulting in a much more gradual rise and drop in levels. This helps to control blood sugars, energy level, and cravings and can assist in attempts to lose weight.

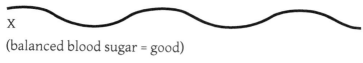

X

(balanced blood sugar = good)

The other thing to consider in balancing blood sugars is caffeine. On its own, caffeine does not directly increase blood sugar; it's often the milk, cream, or sugar that does that. However, indirectly, caffeine does have an impact on blood sugars. Having a cup of coffee first thing in the morning is sort of like a hit to your adrenal glands, telling them, "Hey, wake up, we're being chased by a lion!"

Of course, there is no lion, but your body doesn't know this. Instead, it thinks about the request and realizes that you've been sleeping all night and have no quick energy to access to run away. That's where your liver pipes in and says, "Hey, guys, I can help! I've got some sugar stored over here." So it kicks out some stored sugar (glucose), which helps your body run away from the lion. But there is no lion. So your muscles don't use up that sugar floating around, and it ends up causing insulin to be released, which increases the storage of fat. This propels that sugar crash-and-burn cycle, even in people who don't eat breakfast. I'm not sure that everyone needs to give up their morning cup of java, but you should at least put some protein in your body first to help balance blood sugars for the day.

That covers breakfast, but what about the rest of the day? In the next chapter, The Optimal Portion Plate, we'll explore *what* you should be eating throughout the day and *how much*.

Chapter Seven

The Optimal Portion Plate

There are several ways to fill a plate, and the responsibility of what goes on it is completely up to you. Despite suggesting what you should do, I can't make you do it. If you want to be healthy, then you should eat mostly healthy foods, no exceptions.

Remember, the nutrients that your body needs (water, vitamins, minerals, protein, carbohydrates, and fats) are the foods that should go on your plate. By identifying what your goals are, you will have more motivation to make changes than you will if someone simply tells you what to eat for every meal.

For most people, their primary goal is to lose weight. With that goal in mind, think about each food item before it goes on your plate and ask, "Will eating this item help me achieve my goal of weight loss? Or will it hurt me and add to my current weight?" Even people with a very basic level of nutrition can grasp this concept. Eating highly refined foods such as soda pop, chips, cookies, and crackers will sabotage weight loss goals, even if they are "oh-so delicious!"

Plate Size

First off, the average plate size is way too big. Brian Wansink, Director of the Cornell Food and Brand Lab, stated that between 1900 and 2010, the size of dinner plates increased from 9.6 inches to 11.8 inches, which is almost 23 percent. This increase in size results in the over-serving of food. Essentially, the larger your plate, the more you'll put on it. The relationship between plate size and the amount of food you put on it is called the Delboeuf illusion.

Just in case you think you are well-educated enough not to make the mistake of over-serving yourself when you have a bigger plate, think again. Studies show that even nutrition experts and nutrition graduate students make this same mistake unless they are being extremely vigilant! These are the people who should "know better," but they are just as predisposed to the same bias as you. It goes to show how powerful our minds can be—even if you think you are one of the special few to be the exception to this rule!

There is an upside to this illusion. This same powerful relationship with our plate size can be used to our advantage. When we have a smaller plate size, thanks to that same serving bias, we tend to under-serve ourselves. This is because we perceive the portion to be larger than it is, because proportionately, the same serving size looks bigger on a smaller plate. What's the takeaway message? Use smaller plates if you are trying to cut back on your calories.

Another way of cutting back on calories can be done by simply changing the color of your plate or tablecloth. The Delboeuf illusion shows that we have a greater bias when there is a greater color contrast between our food and our plates or tablecloths. Want to eat even smaller portions? Put your pale-colored food on a small, dark plate, and your dark-colored food on a small, white plate.

Easy and effortless "food hacks" like this can also help us eat more of the foods that are healthier for us, such as vegetables, which most people generally don't eat enough of. By using a larger plate or bowl for your salad, you will subconsciously fill it with more than you would if it were

a smaller size. This allows you to eat more vegetables without any extra effort. Put your dark green veggies on a large, black plate, and you'll be eating more of them without even realizing it.

What to Put on That Plate

While it's impossible to come up with a one-size-fits-all approach to eating, it's not impossible to create a healthy starting point that can be modified to suit your needs. I've looked at a lot of the basic nutrition recommendations and have come up with a modified version of the portion plate because it does help you to learn how to balance portions.

These recommendations have been compiled from existing literature on disease prevention, health promotion, and nutrition courses that promote optimal health. The suggestions consider which foods are linked to cancer, diabetes, weight gain, cholesterol, and blood pressure issues, and suggest to reduce or eliminate certain foods. At the same time, my optimal portion plate encourages the consumption of unprocessed, unrefined foods with higher nutrition density, as they are linked to healthy benefits. If you've seen a portion plate concept before, don't skip ahead—I suggest tips that are different than anything you've probably seen before, and they have resulted in big changes for my clients. The optimal nutrition plate is designed to help you **thrive**, not to simply **survive**, as many other food guides propose.

Dave came to see me for some nutrition advice to help improve his blood test results. He had slightly elevated blood sugar and cholesterol, his blood pressure was borderline, and he was about 40 pounds overweight. Overall, Dave thought he was a pretty healthy guy and was surprised that his lab results showed any problems. Being a top manager in his engineering firm, Dave was a busy guy and wanted to get in and out of the appointment as quickly as possible. He wanted a copy of a diet to fix his problems and the exact number of calories he should consume in a day so that he could track it on his phone.

Dave's story isn't unique. Lots of people come in wanting a quick, easy fix and a specific, detailed plan that they can follow verbatim to get back on track as quickly as possible. In the real world, it doesn't work that way, and anyone who does provide meal plan templates should recognize that those plans aren't customized to clients' individual needs.

The most important thing to realize is that the portion plate concept is only a starting **template** and does not need to be executed in the exact ratios shown in order to achieve results. In fact, I'd like you to make notes on it to make it unique for your situation. As long as you have valid reasons for why you are making different food choices or adjusting the recommendations (e.g., allergies, cultural beliefs, activity level), you will be moving in the right direction. Adjusting the proportions on the plate may also be necessary for certain conditions. For example, people with gastrointestinal concerns (Crohn's, colitis, IBS, etc.) may not be able to start with a half a plate of vegetables due to side effects such as gas and bloating. Over time, with a structured plan, they may be able to increase their consumption of vegetables.

Similarly, you are able to alter the optimal portion plate to fit the specific diet that you want to follow. Like the paleo approach? Eliminate the foods listed in the processed sections of proteins and carbohydrates along with all grains and tubers. Want to go vegan? Choose high-quality vegetarian protein sources like beans, lentils, and whole soybeans and avoid all those processed vegan meats that are full of unnecessary chemicals. It doesn't really matter if you are on a strict autoimmune protocol diet, FODMAP-free, nightshade-free, or if you don't have a clue what those terms mean. Starting with a healthy foundation of mostly unprocessed foods is always a great place to start to get healthier.

Another example of when to vary the portions on the plate would be if you are trying to lose a large amount of weight. You'll likely want to increase protein and decrease carbohydrates while maintaining a high intake of vegetables and fiber. There are numerous other conditions to consider, and it would be impossible to give specific examples of every possible modification. However, you can customize these recommendations to fit your specific needs.

Please recognize that the foods listed in each part of the plate are examples only. There are many other foods available, and again, it would

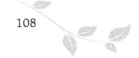

The Optimal Nutrition Plate

Focus on quality, not calories
Eat mostly fresh, unprocessed, unpackaged, organic/pastured/grass-fed foods that are in their most natural state

NON-STARCHY VEGETABLES
-Fiber, vitamins, minerals, antioxidants, phytonutrients
-Should make up half of your meal/snack
-**Size**: approximately two handfuls

Eat all different colors: red, orange, yellow, green, purple, white

Some examples:
Herbs: cilantro, mint, parsley
Greens: arugula, cabbage, chard, collards, kale, lettuce, mustard greens, spinach
Squash: acorn, butternut, delicata, spaghetti squash, zucchini
Bulbs: garlic, leek, onion
Cruciferous: broccoli, cabbage, cauliflower
Other: celery, cucumber, eggplant, mushrooms, peas, peppers, tomato

HEALTHY FATS**
-Build your immune system, part of brain and hormone production, keep hair/nails healthy
-Avocados/acovado oil, coconut, nuts/nut butters, olives/olive oil, seeds

FIBER
-Keeps the trains running on time, eliminates some toxins and cholesterol
-Chia seed, flax seed (ground), hemp seed
-Supplements: Benefiber, Metamucil

THIRSTY?
-Drink water or herbal tea
-0.2–0.5 oz/lb body weight

PROTEIN
-Building block for muscle mass, regulate blood sugar, help keep you feeling full longer, help with weight loss
-Should make up one-fourth of your meal/snack
-**Size**: approximately the palm of your hand

Some examples:
Meat: beef, bison, boar, buffalo, goat, pork
Poultry: chicken, duck, eggs, goose, pheasant, turkey
Fish: salmon, tuna, snapper, swordfish
Seafood/Shellfish: clams, crab, lobster, mussels, oysters, shrimp
Alternatives: beans, edamame, hemp/pea protein, legumes, lentils, nuts, tempeh, tofu

Reduce or eliminate:
Processed Foods: bacon/turkey bacon, cheese, deli meats, sausage, TVP, veggie ground round
CAFO/Conventionally raised meats

CARBOHYDRATES (Sugar*)
-Turn into sugar to provide the body with energy
-Should make up one-fourth of your meal/snack or less
-**Size**: one small fist (15 g per serving) Total less than 130 g per day
-Recommended servings:

Some examples:
Fruit: fresh
Starchy/root veggies: beet, carrot, corn, potato, sweet potato, yam, yucca
Dairy: milk, yogurt
Whole grains: amaranth, barley, buckwheat, quinoa, rice (brown/wild), whole oats (half cup cooked grains = one serving)

Reduce or eliminate:
Processed foods: bagels, bread, cereal, chips, cookies, crackers, quick oatmeal, pasta, pitas, tortillas
Fruit: canned, dried, packaged
Drinks: pop, juice
Sugar/candy/ice cream

*Eat all carbs with some type of protein to slow the digestion of sugars
**Caffeine may raise blood sugar

be impossible to list every vegetable, protein, and carbohydrate on one page. If you don't like the examples listed, don't obsess over it and feel that you need to eat them. Try other foods and experiment with ones you've never tried before.

What's on the Optimal Portion Plate?

Life would be easier for health care professionals if there was one perfect recommendation we could give to all of their patients. Unfortunately, as I've already mentioned, this doesn't work. This makes it difficult because, as a result, health care pros like me feel like we need to keep five or ten or twenty different diet plans on hand for all of our different types of patients. The "optimal portion plate" gives us the best of both worlds—one easy-to-use handout that's adaptable to any diet or medical condition.

Looking at what's on your plate, it's going to vary a bit from someone else, and that's okay. We don't all have to eat exactly the same. The optimal portion plate should be looked at as a template that can be modified for your unique situation. When you look at a traditional portion plate, it's built with half the plate as vegetables, one-quarter protein, and one-quarter starch with a glass of milk and a fruit at every meal. In my experience, that's far too many carbohydrates for most people. Read on to find out why!

Carbohydrates

For both carbohydrates and proteins, I've separated whole foods from processed foods. Processed foods are connected to cancer, chronic diseases, and weight gain and should be reduced or completely eliminated from your diet due to their health risks. If you have chronic diseases, it's in your best interest to completely stop eating these foods, even though you might like them. If you are healthier, you may be able to get away with the occasional indulgence without too much impact on your health. To reach *optimal health*, you may want to completely avoid these foods.

It's quiz time! Remember in the nutrition introduction, when I mentioned that I was going to test you on how carbohydrates break down? What types of carbohydrates turn into sugar?

Give up?

All carbohydrates, regardless of whether they are healthy or not, turn into sugar in the body! Yes, **all** of them (except fiber)! This is a really frustrating topic to discuss with clients because nutrition labeling has confused or misled most people into false beliefs about carbohydrates.

Ronald, a sixty-four-year-old obese man with type two diabetes, told me that he's been eating crackers and chips because they have zero grams of sugar and are okay to eat with his condition. What he's not looking at are the total grams of carbohydrates listed on the label above the sugar line.

It's quite common to find foods that have *zero grams of sugar* listed but are still extremely high in *total carbohydrates*. These carbohydrates still turn into sugar in the body, which sets off that volatile up and down blood sugar curve we looked at earlier. This is where people's heads usually start to spin, as they learn how many foods turn into sugar. Foods like fruit, starchy root vegetables like potatoes, sweet potatoes, beets and carrots, and whole grains—all turn into sugar. Most people don't realize that milk and yogurt turn into sugar. Even though they have some protein, they have lots of carbohydrates, too.

Not everyone needs to eliminate carbohydrate-based foods; in fact, I'd advise against it. You need some carbohydrates to run your engine. What you don't need is a giant sugar bomb first thing in the morning, which is the part of the plate where most breakfasts live. Imagine a healthy breakfast of yogurt, fruit, and granola. On paper, this appears to be a healthy, nutritious breakfast. However, it's far from being *balanced*. All of these foods contain carbohydrates that break down into sugar, with little protein or fiber to balance out the sharp rise in blood sugar that you will get from this sugar bomb.

Dena almost broke down into tears when she found out how much sugar she was eating by having fruit, yogurt, and granola for breakfast, stating, "But I thought I was eating healthy!" It's not that she's eating *unhealthy.* Dena is eating *imbalanced*, which is totally different. When eating foods that balance blood sugar, you can lose weight faster, balance blood sugars more efficiently with less medication, and get better body composition changes. Foods can be healthy, but that doesn't make them right for every person.

The carbohydrates you definitely want to reduce or eliminate are ones that are processed and highly refined. These include breads, pasta, chips, crackers, popcorn, bagels, quick oatmeal, tortillas, pita breads, canned fruit, pop, juice, and candy.

Protein

As we've previously discussed, protein foods break down into amino acids, which are the building blocks of muscle mass. They also regulate blood sugar and keep you feeling fuller longer. An easy way to measure a protein serving is to make it the size of the palm of your hand. Your hand might be larger or smaller than someone else's, but it's in proportion to your body size, which helps to keep the portion size more appropriate for you. The bigger the person, the more protein is needed to support your muscle mass.

Several studies support the effectiveness of increased protein consumption during weight loss, as it helps prevent the loss of muscle mass that commonly occurs, and because of its satiating properties. Protein can be consumed as different types of meat, poultry, fish, and eggs and can also be found in incomplete sources of protein such as beans, legumes, and nuts. You'll want to cut back on the processed sources of protein like protein powders, texturized vegetable protein, vegetarian "meats," deli meats, sausage, and cheese. These foods should be viewed more as condiments and eaten sparingly.

Carla, a lean and healthy mom in her forties, came to me with extremely high LDL cholesterol. She ate healthy, exercised, had little stress, slept well, and had no family history of high cholesterol. There was no reason for her to have high cholesterol, yet she did. After taking a diet history, I noticed that Carla had cheese at almost every meal in some form

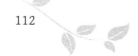

or another. She was using cheese as her main protein source and often ate cheese and crackers after work, another high source of bad fat.

After working with Carla for only three months and encouraging her to reduce cheese to only a few times per month, she was able to return her cholesterol to a normal level. She made no other diet or lifestyle changes to create this improvement. Diet is an incredibly powerful way to improve your health!

Vegetables

Vegetables are vital for a variety of reasons. Vegetables help introduce a variety of vitamins, minerals, antioxidants (powerful baskets that scoop the bad stuff out of your body), phytonutrients (plant-based nutrients), and fiber. It's important to eat a large variety of vegetables in order to take on a wide variety of nutrients.

Eat from the rainbow—consume red, yellow, orange, purple, and white vegetables, as they all have different health properties. As a side note, people tell me all the time that they've heard there is no nutritional value in white foods, so they don't eat white vegetables. But by cutting out the white foods, you are losing great nutrients from foods like garlic, ginger, onions, and mushrooms that have several known health properties. Just because a vegetable doesn't have a vibrant color doesn't mean that it's not nutritious. Within the different colors, you'll want to get a wide variety of different types of vegetables such as squash, herbs, greens, bulbs, cruciferous vegetables, and nightshades.

Initially, you'll want to get those veggies in your body any way you can. Eat them however you want: boiled, baked, steamed, sautéed, barbecued, or raw. At first, your primary goal is to just get them *in*! One serving of a leafy vegetable is about two handfuls, and most other veggies are about one cup in size.

Be careful about how you introduce vegetables into your diet. If you aren't used to eating *any* vegetables and suddenly start eating half a plate of raw cruciferous vegetables at every meal, you will likely end up with GI symptoms like gas, bloating, or diarrhea. This negative feedback is telling you to stop eating all of this healthy fiber, and you'll likely swear off vegetables for the rest of your life. That's not my goal!

Start introducing vegetables slowly and increase servings gradually as you become better able to digest them. The goal should be to get up to half a plate, three times a day over the course of three months, six months, or even a year for people with known digestive difficulties like Crohn's, colitis, diverticulitis, diverticulosis, and celiac disease. People with those medical conditions may need to introduce their foods even more slowly or modify the way they eat vegetables to reduce the fiber content.

You can modify vegetables by juicing or blending them so that you can get the nutritional value of the vegetable without the fiber that is often problematic. Other tips are to chop the veggies finely and cook them until they fall apart to make them more digestible. Initially, this will likely reduce the nutrition content of the vegetable, as boiling chopped vegetables until they are mushy will likely destroy a significant part of the nutrition, especially if the water is discarded. However, by making the vegetable more digestible, you may actually absorb a small amount—let's say 10 percent—of the total nutritional value. While far from optimal, this is better than 100 percent of the nutritional value of a raw food passing straight through your digestive tract and not getting absorbed at all.

Over time, as you tolerate the well-cooked foods better and no longer have symptoms of gas, bloating, or diarrhea after eating them, slowly cut back on the cooking time by a few minutes every few days or weeks. For example, instead of boiling cauliflower for thirty minutes, you could reduce the cook time to twenty-eight minutes and see how your digestion changes. Over time, this method will help slowly increase your tolerance to vegetables and will help you extract more nutrition from your food.

Fats

You'll notice that fat isn't specifically on the portion plate, and that's intentional. These requirements vary significantly for different people. The emphasis here should be on high-quality fats. That means fats that have less refining done to them to make them edible, such as avocados, coconuts, nuts, and seeds. You'll want to use caution if you cook with

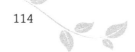

fats, as some of them, such as olive oil, turn rancid with exposure to heat. These heat-sensitive fats should be used as toppings for vegetables or salads, and other more stable fats such as coconut, avocado, or grapeseed oil should be used for cooking. Choose quality over quantity!

Fiber

As a whole, most of us don't come anywhere close to our recommended daily intake of fiber, so that's another area of nutrition where we are failing miserably. Most people get fewer than 10 grams of fiber each day. The recommendations for adult men sit at 38 grams and 25 grams for adult women, much higher than most of us get.

Fiber is a great way to "keep the trains running on time." Yup, I'm talking about pooping! Fiber adds bulk to the stool—or bowel movement or whatever other "nice" name you have for your poo. It also lowers cholesterol and balances blood sugar. The mistake that most people make is to add a ton of fiber into their diet with no other changes, and then they end up constipated.

Think of fiber like concrete. The right amount, mixed with water, will create a few nicely formed bricks. Too much concrete, without enough water, and you'll end up with one giant rock inside your intestines. For extra fiber, you can add whole foods like vegetables, chia seed, ground flax seed, hemp seed, inulin or psyllium husk, or supplements like Benefiber that have few added chemicals. Just make sure you add extra water to your diet to help "thin" the fiber so it doesn't plug up the pipes.

Water

You'll want to drink enough water or decaffeinated beverages like caffeine-free tea in order to stay hydrated and to flush the toxins out of your body. Some people can drink fewer fluids by compensating with a diet rich in hydrated foods like vegetables and fruits, but they will generally have a low sweat rate or live in a cool climate. Those who should drink more fluids include people with inflammatory issues, people who need to improve their detoxification process, or people who need to lose weight. Those who should drink more fluids tend to be active, live in hotter climates, or eat a lot of dry, processed foods. Remember that to be at a more ideal hydration status, your pee should be clear or lightly colored.

Balancing Specific Meals

I've frequently been asked about how to apply the optimal portion plate to breakfast because so many people are used to eating primarily carbohydrate-rich foods in the morning. The concept of having a salad for breakfast isn't appealing, and most people's minds draw a blank when considering other options for breakfast foods.

A great breakfast option is an omelet that you can bake ahead of time. Sauté four or five cups of fresh, seasonal vegetables until the water just starts to get released, and then dump them in a lasagna pan without the liquids. I typically put in vegetables I don't munch on as snacks, such as leeks or onions, mushrooms, and spinach because they cook up really nicely. Then scramble a dozen eggs and pour them on top of the vegetables. It takes about thirty minutes to bake and can easily be done when you are making Sunday-night dinner. That gives you eight large pieces of healthy omelet that can be portioned out for the week. I've even had clients freeze portions for later.

Another option would be to make a breakfast hash with grated potato or sweet potato with and an equal amount of lean ground chicken, turkey, or pork. I love adding cinnamon and mild curry powder with it, but you can add whatever herbs and spices you like. If you feel like adding some veggies, you can add mushrooms, onions, or peppers (or anything else you like) to increase the nutritional value. If you don't want to eat any veggies at breakfast, at least the protein and carbohydrates are balanced.

If you are resistant to eating vegetables at breakfast, consider a veggie smoothie made with water and one serving of fruit. Drink it while you are eating some protein like a boiled egg, some salmon, or a lean breakfast patty made from lean ground meat. Be creative.

It's easier to apply the concept of balance to lunches and dinners, as you are likely much more comfortable with eating vegetables, protein,

and carbohydrates for those meals. It's often just the portion size that needs to be adjusted. Most commonly, you will need to cut back on your carbohydrates and increase your vegetable intake. If you are trying to lose weight, I'd also suggest eliminating all liquid calories, as it's much easier to drink calories than it is to eat them. This can be used in reverse if you are a hard gainer (someone who has a hard time putting on weight).

How to Eat

We've all grown up eating, but most of us were likely never taught how to truly eat properly. To help get even more benefits from the portion plate, here are a few more tips on how to eat properly.

- It takes at least twenty minutes to feel full. Eat until you are comfortably full, not stuffed.
  - ▷ Eating slowly allows this normal feedback mechanism to kick in, telling the body to stop eating before it's overfilled.
- Chew your food thoroughly.
  - ▷ This helps break your food down into smaller pieces, mixes saliva into them, and initiates the breakdown process where it's meant to start.
- Chew liquid foods.
  - ▷ Even liquid calories need to have saliva mixed into them to break them down properly.
- Eat mindfully.
  - ▷ What does your food smell like?
  - ▷ What does your food taste like?
  - ▷ What is the texture of your food?
  - ▷ What temperature is your food?
  - ▷ What does your food look like?
- Eat enough calories to support your activity level.
  - ▷ Most people overestimate the number of calories they burn and underestimate the amount they consume. Use this knowledge to your advantage! Reduce carbohydrate-dense foods if you are inactive or have a low activity level.

Chapter Eight

False Beliefs About Food

*W*e all have stories that we tell ourselves about food. The problem with this is that often, what we repeat to ourselves over and over again tends to become our reality, making our belief even stronger.

Aleksandra grew up in a traditional Ukrainian household where she was told that she was big-boned. She wasn't allowed to leave the table until all the food was gone because her mother told her, "I've slaved over the stove all day to make you good food. You can't waste it." Aleksandra believed she was showing her love for her mom by eating whatever food was put in front of her, even though she wasn't happy with her waistline. As an adult, Aleksandra struggled even more with her weight and was unable to lose the additional fifty pounds that she put on with her third pregnancy. Aleksandra was frustrated about not being able to lose weight but couldn't bear to cut back on her food portions because she was worried her mom wouldn't feel loved.

Aleksandra's story is all too common. I could probably write a whole book on the stories I've heard people tell themselves about food. Often, those stories aren't even true, and to achieve optimal health, they need to be changed.

The best way to make a lasting change is to evaluate your current belief and really analyze if you still believe it to be true. Some of our beliefs come from what our parents told us while we were growing up. Some of them come from the marketing that we are constantly bombarded with in the media. Other beliefs are based on misinterpreting information, lack of education or knowledge, or peers who pass on their personal beliefs. Regardless of how we have acquired our beliefs, we are able to change them if we really want to.

In the following section, I've listed some of the most common examples of food beliefs. These are important for you to examine in order to be more successful in achieving long-lasting results.

Making bad food choices is "cheating"

There's a reason that most people feel compelled to "cheat" on their nutritional choices even when they're committed to making healthy changes. Humans are naturally drawn to enjoy foods that are sweet or fatty because those foods tend to be calorie-dense. Calorie-dense food kept us alive in times of famine thousands of years ago. Now, we have much more accessibility to those calorie-rich foods, but that same regulatory system hasn't turned off.

I teach my clients to change their language about food—to get rid of words like "cheat," "being good," or "being bad." You are simply making a choice. It's either a more nutritious choice or a less nutritious choice. It's a choice, not a cheat. When you can get rid of the guilt that comes from cheating, you are able to be much more successful in sticking with food choices. Keep reading, and I'll give you three key questions to ask yourself before making food choices.

You can negate the impact of bad food choices

Many people feel that they can eat good food to counter the effects of bad food. Gerry firmly believed that he could eat a chocolate bar as an afternoon snack because he always ate a large salad at lunch—as if the good salad canceled out the bad chocolate bar. Unfortunately, we are not able to cancel out the negative effects of one type of food by eating something

else. Yes, the salad was a fantastic choice and provided Gerry's body with many vitamins and minerals, but it didn't undo the impact that the sugar in the chocolate bar had on his hormones or insulin release. The calories might balance out at the end of the day, but the health impact may not.

In another example, Lynda was obese, weighing more than 400 pounds. She was on a mission to lose weight and get healthy again. She cut down her intake to 2,000 calories each day and started working out. However, Lynda figured that by exercising and burning 500 calories each day, it meant she could eat an extra 500 calories because they were just a wash. So, despite telling me that she was eating 2,000 calories a day, she was actually eating 2,500 calories, which is a whole different story. Most fitness calculators overestimate calories burned and underestimate the calories consumed to begin with, leading to much slower weight loss than anticipated. No wonder she had only lost four and a half pounds over two months.

Vegetables are boring and taste bland

Eating vegetables doesn't have to be boring or tasteless. Start with eating the best quality and freshest vegetables you can afford, and the taste will dramatically improve. If you grow your own veggies, nothing beats the taste of a fresh garden carrot or tomato. Make sure that you use compost and keep your soil healthy so that it's full of nutrients for years to come.

When veggies don't taste great on their own, or their taste isn't to your palate, add additional herbs and spices to add flavor without adding calories. There are literally hundreds of spices out there—if you ate a carrot with only one new spice on it each day, you could eat carrots with hundreds of different flavors. People who are bored with their food need to be more creative and resourceful. Look up new recipes—there are millions of them available for free online!

It's up to the method to change your habit

I can't count the number of times I've heard someone say that they've tried every diet imaginable, and none of them worked. Of course they didn't work—those methods are faulty!

We live in a society that cultivates a lack of personal responsibility. It's not your fault. It's the method. You need to accept that change can be uncomfortable. Despite not liking the feeling of being uncomfortable, you need to get through that in order to truly see change. Sometimes, you just need to rip off the band-aid. Other times, you need to peel it back slowly. Either way, it needs to come off, or you'll end up with one nasty infection underneath.

Short-term diets lead to a lifetime of frustration. It's better to *permanently* change. Stop dieting and start making permanent dietary changes today.

You can be good 80 percent of the time and cheat 20 percent of the time

Ah, the good old 80/20 rule. As the saying goes, "If you eat good food 80 percent of the time, then 20 percent of the time, you can afford to eat whatever you want." Unfortunately, there are a few inherent flaws with that philosophy.

First of all, most people who subscribe to this method end up eating way more than 20 percent of their calories from poor-quality nutritional choices. For example, in a typical day, Trina had a large vanilla latte and a blueberry muffin for breakfast, a granola bar for an afternoon snack, and a light beer with dinner. On their own, each of these items doesn't seem like much, so most people don't think twice about eating them. But when you add up the caloric content from that latte, muffin, granola bar, and beer, it makes up an extra 870 calories that weren't even accounted for. Being on a typical 2,000-calorie per day diet means that Trina's eating 43.5 percent of her calories from junk food. That's almost half of her daily calories, which is far from "being bad" only 20 percent of the time. Plus, these types of food choices commonly contain a lot of sugar, processed grains, and preservatives, and aren't adding much to meet normal daily nutritional requirements, let alone *optimal* nutrition requirements.

The second downfall of the 80/20 rule is that many individuals become so fixated on the 20 percent that they plan their weeks just waiting for their "cheat" meal. They get so fixated with the 20 percent that they

can't even enjoy the other 80 percent of their diet. It makes the other foods taste less appealing because, heck, they're only veggies. Whatever happened to enjoying fresh, raw food right out of the garden?

The third flaw with the 80/20 rule is that it doesn't work for everyone. For some people to be healthy, they might need a ratio of 95/5. Or someone who has really good genetics and is much hardier may be able to get away with a 70/30 ratio. You'll want to consider your current health status, health and fitness goals, need for mental clarity, medical conditions, allergies or food intolerances, stress level, and sleep. Your ratio will likely change over time as you change jobs, have higher or lower stress, and are more or less active. It will also change with age and a number of other lifestyle factors.

Put simply, if you want to get 80 percent results, then eat well 80 percent of the time. If you want to achieve optimal results, you'll likely want to be closer to 100 percent. No one should become so obsessive over food that there is no wiggle room to play with (unless it's an allergy), but don't use silly rules to justify eating junk. If you want better health, eat better foods most of the time.

Calories in equals calories out

Not all calories are equal. The number of calories does matter, but the number is not the only part of nutrition that should be considered. People think that if they burn 1,000 calories, they can eat 1,000 calories, but that math seldom adds up. You need to look at the *quality* of the calories to determine how they affect the body.

I'll give you an extreme example of why calories are not equal. Let's compare two servings of foods that are both 1,000 calories. On paper, 1,000 calories of spinach and 1,000 calories of chocolate are equal. In reality, they are far from equal. For starters, the portion size is significantly different. The chocolate works out to be about forty-five pieces. You could easily eat that in one sitting. You may not feel good after eating that much chocolate, but you *could* physically do it. In comparison, 1,000 calories of raw spinach works out to 144 cups. Now, if you sat down in the kitchen with your whole family, it's unlikely that you'd be able to eat 144 cups of spinach over the course of an entire day, let alone in one sitting.

Those foods also have very different nutrient profiles. The chocolate has much more fat and carbohydrates and little fiber or nutrients. In comparison, the spinach shockingly has much more protein and is higher in fiber, vitamins, minerals, and phytonutrients. It's also important to look at the impact on insulin and blood sugar that these two foods have. With the chocolate having a whopping 115 grams of sugar, the pancreas is going to have to work double time to produce enough insulin to deal with that sugar. The spinach will cause a much slower rise in blood sugar, with only 9 grams of sugar. Plus, it will take far longer for that sugar to get into the body because it would be impossible to eat all of the spinach in the same timeframe as the chocolate. The fiber in the spinach would also slow the rate of carbohydrate breakdown.

	Milk Chocolate	Raw Spinach
Calories	1000	1000
Serving size	45 pieces	144 cups
Protein	15	62
Carbohydrates	125	78
Fiber	5	48
Sugar	115	9
Fat	60	8
Saturated Fat	35	1
Polyunsaturated Fat	0	4
Cholesterol	50	0
Vitamin A	0	4051
Vitamin C	0	1012
Calcium	40	214
Iron	10	325

* Source: My Fitness Pal

I don't have time to eat healthy

I regularly hear excuses from patients that they don't have time to eat healthy. My response: You don't have time to not eat healthy! You are only given a short time on this Earth, and you are only given one body to do it. By eating healthy most of the time, you will keep your body in better shape and be able to do more with it.

Olga came in to see me, walking slowly with her walker and barely able to get in and out of the chair in my office. She asked me where she could get some "new parts" from. The body shop down the street was offering new parts, and she wanted some. New hips. New knees. New pancreas.

Unfortunately, it doesn't work that way. We can't just go to a body shop to get new parts. By taking care of your "parts" in the first place, you'll be able to keep them in working order longer than if you neglect them.

Other thoughts on dietary choices and cheating

Why do we feel we need to cheat in the first place? What is the point of a cheat? A mental break? Sometimes, you just need to give yourself permission to make less nutrient-dense choices. It's not about perfection. It's also not about being a "good" person or a "bad" person because of the choices you make. Food choices don't make you good or bad. They are simply choices.

Chapter Nine

Why Do You Eat?

*L*et's look at the core foundation of eating. There are several reasons why you eat, but there truly is only one reason why you need to eat, and that is survival. You *need* to eat to fuel your body, to keep your engine running—you do not *need* to eat a double-stuffed, deep-fried cookie coated in chocolate, regardless of how much you might tell yourself that you might die if you don't.

Overall, you only need to eat to provide your body with nutrients, and you only need to drink water to keep your cells hydrated. Without these essential nutrients in balance, our bodies do not function optimally and may shut down or experience negative effects over time.

Despite only needing to eat for one reason, we do end up eating for other reasons, most of which are tied to our culture or our emotions. We eat during different occasions such as birthdays, anniversaries, holidays, or other celebrations. Food has a way of bringing cultures together. It has religious significance—the breaking of bread or sharing of a sacred cup of wine with our families or communities. We have food at weddings and at funerals. We use eating as an excuse to get together with friends: "Let's go out for breakfast together and catch up." We eat or drink because of work functions: "I have a business meeting this afternoon, and we're going out for drinks with the guys after to debrief," or "I'm going to a business lunch."

We also eat for many emotional reasons. We often end up eating because of peer pressure because everyone else is eating something. It's someone's birthday at work, and the cake is being passed around the boardroom. You don't want to be the only person left out. People might wonder why you aren't eating it. Maybe a coworker of yours made it from scratch, and you don't want to offend her hard work. It might hurt her feelings not to eat it, and you'll feel guilty. Plus, it looks so delicious, and you've been good on your diet all week. And you deserve a treat, it's been a tough day. . . .

A common guilt trap is when you are over at your parents' house for Christmas dinner. Your mom has slaved over the stove all day preparing all of the foods that she thinks you love. You've already eaten an entire plate and are feeling full. Mom says, "There's just a little bit more. Why don't you finish it off?" Mom went through all this trouble to prepare your favorite foods, and you don't want to disappoint her. So you go back for a second helping and finish off what's on the table, now feeling even fuller. But wait! There's still dessert. And who could resist mom's famous dessert? So you eat even more and finish dinner feeling uncomfortably bloated and frustrated with yourself for eating too much. Sound familiar?

We eat for other reasons, too. We eat out of boredom. We eat because it's lunchtime and this is "the only time I have to eat before I'm off work at the end of the day." We eat because of cravings. We eat when we are excited. We eat to celebrate. We eat because we are sad. We eat because it's a holiday. We eat because it's pizza Friday. We eat because it's . . . Tuesday—the list could go on and on. I have even witnessed a coworker, Jan, having conversations with her food: "What's that, little chocolate? You want me to eat you? Oh, you do? Okay! Come jump into my mouth. . . . Oh . . . you taste delicious. See? You made me eat you. I couldn't help it!"

Food does not have a voice. It is not a person. It should not have power over us, and yet, for some people, it does. This is called an *associative food craving*. It happens when we associate certain events with certain foods. Common examples of these types of cravings are movies

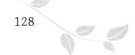

and popcorn, coffee with breakfast, or snacking at your desk. We can also associate certain feelings with food choices; when we are sad, we eat junk food, or when we are happy, we drink wine. The more often we indulge in these associations, the stronger they get, to the point that we aren't even consciously aware of them.

I work with my clients to help cut down on the emotional connections they have with food. I don't know if it's ever possible to cut out these connections completely, but we can reduce the emotional connection.

There are three simple questions I started asking my clients back when I was a personal trainer, and I've had such good success with them that I've kept it as part of my practice for well over a decade. By being more mindful of *why* we are eating, we are able to take back control over our impulses. We regain power over food, instead of food having power over us.

At first, this exercise may seem challenging. You might even forget to do this activity and then remember only after you've eaten the food. Don't beat yourself up if you recognize that you ate something impulsively. This awareness will help you make better decisions next time. Ask yourself the following questions every time you think about eating or drinking something.

1. Why am I eating this food?

You can eat more or less food to control your body weight, or you can change the types of food that you are eating to affect your body composition. So the first question to ask yourself is, "Why am I eating this food?"

As I've already reviewed, the only reason you need to eat is to fuel your body or rehydrate, but we know that survival isn't generally *why* we eat. There are many different reasons (I've already mentioned some of them, but maybe you have a different reason that I haven't even touched on).

When you sit down to enjoy a snack or a meal, think about the reason why you are eating or drinking. Now that you have an answer, make sure you are honest with yourself. Ask yourself, "Is this the right reason for me to eat right now?" Maybe yes, and maybe no. Just because everyone else is eating does not mean that it's right for you. You have different goals and priorities than other people, and you need to decide if you are eating for the right reasons.

If you can't come up with a reason that you feel good about, then you shouldn't be eating that food. This is when it's important to really be honest with yourself.

2. How will this food make me feel when I eat it?

The second question to ask is, "How will this food make me feel when I eat it?" I usually get a variety of answers when I ask this one. Sometimes, people are so unaware of their bodies that their only answer is "fine. . . ." Once they start paying closer attention, however, they may start to notice other feelings.

Some of my clients report feeling bloated from eating certain foods but not from eating others. Or having increased or decreased energy, or feeling foggy-headed, jittery, irritable, or even depressed. Some people feel good about themselves for making healthy choices but beat themselves up for making bad choices. Many of my clients will tell me that they are excited to eat junk food, but then secretly beat themselves up inside after they've eaten it because they feel so guilty.

Generally, you want to eat foods that make you feel good—foods that make you feel energized, healthy, strong and clear-minded. Make sure that you are telling yourself the truth!

3. Will eating this food help me achieve my goal?

The last question to ask is, "Will eating this food help me achieve my health/weight loss goals?" This one has a pretty straightforward answer. It's either yes or no.

You can't really beat around the bush on this one, and it's best if you tell yourself the truth instead of making up silly rules. I've heard clients tell me jokingly that "calories don't count on your birthday," or that "cookies don't have calories if they are broken in half." Another classic: "If no one saw you eat it, it doesn't count."

Even if these rules are just jokes, they're still flat-out lies. Your food choice is either going to help you accomplish your health goal or it isn't. Black or white. Yes or no.

To achieve optimal health, the answers to these three questions do not always need to be perfect. Suppose that tomorrow is your birthday, and you want to have a piece of cake. Are you eating the cake for its high nutritional value? Probably not. Will it make you feel good eating it? Perhaps, but not necessarily. And will eating birthday cake help you lose weight? Definitely not. However, it's your birthday, and you've decided that you want to have a piece of cake, and that's okay. Have your cake, eat it slowly so that you enjoy it, and then move on.

What I encourage my clients to do is to mostly eat foods for the right reasons (hungry, need fuel, good nutrition, etc.), that make them feel good and give them energy while working towards achieving their goals. If, every once in a while, their food choices don't line up with these three values, such as on a birthday, that's okay. Try to make food choices that are in line with your goals *more often* than you make choices that go against your goals.

Implementing the Three Questions

You've probably heard that it takes twenty-one days to change a habit and that if you do something for twenty-one days, all your problems will be fixed. From my experience, however, the longer you've had a habit, the longer it will take to change it; it's not tied to a simple twenty-one-day principle.

It does take time to change habits, and practice makes perfect. If you have had bad eating habits for thirty years—or maybe never learned how to eat properly in the first place—you aren't likely to change your habits in just twenty-one days. You'll need to practice over and over until you gain the skills. You will make mistakes. Just pick yourself back up, dust yourself off, and try again. It will get easier to make better choices.

There will be times when food somehow makes its way into your mouth without you even realizing it. In those types of situations, go through the questions after the fact to help learn why you made that choice. Ask yourself, "Why did I eat that food? How do I feel now that I've eaten it? Was that food in line with my goals?"

You'll want to plan your eating around your goals. If your goal is to lose weight, choose foods that are more nutrient-dense and less calorie-dense. If your goal is to gain weight, choose foods that are more calorie-dense.

You'll also want to consider the other key pillars of health and make changes based on those other areas. For example, if you have a strong family history of type two diabetes, are sedentary, or don't sleep well, you likely shouldn't eat carbohydrates with reckless abandon. Consider a more moderate carbohydrate intake to help preserve the function of your pancreas for as long as possible. This would help bring you closer to the concept of optimal health.

The following is a self-reflection activity designed to help you learn more about your food choices. The intent of this information is to build a solid nutritional foundation to positively influence your health.

Thought Changer

1) Why am I eating this food?

....

....

....

2) How will this food make me feel when I eat it?

....

....

....

3) Will eating this food help me achieve my health/weight loss goals?

....

....

....

If you really want to delve deeper into nutrition, here are some other great questions for thinking about food. They should help to shift some of your thoughts around eating habits.

Additional questions to consider

▷ Are you an emotional eater? What emotions make you eat?
▷ How do you use food as a reward?
▷ How do you use food as a crutch?
▷ What are your triggers for overeating? Snacking?
▷ When do you struggle with portion control?
▷ When do you struggle with making good food choices?
▷ Who does the grocery shopping?
▷ Who does the meal planning?
▷ Who does the cooking/food prep?
▷ How many meals per week do you cook?
▷ When and where do you eat?
▷ What else do you do while you are eating? (e.g., drive, watch TV)
▷ What are your favorite foods? How do they make you feel when you eat them?
▷ What times of day do you eat?
▷ How long have you been eating this way?
▷ What will you lose if you give up these foods/this way of eating?
▷ What will you gain if you give up these foods/this way of eating?
▷ What scares you about making a permanent lifestyle change? Is this fear true?
▷ What brings you joy? Happiness? List ideas that aren't related to food.

Motivation for Eating

Generally, most people start their quest to lose weight simply because they want to look better. Some people may consider this to be vanity, but regardless, it can be a pretty powerful motivator.

When we like our appearance more, we feel better about ourselves and, in turn, have better self-esteem. Then we put more effort into keeping our bodies looking better. Conversely, when we feel bad about our bodies, we aren't as motivated to eat good food or to exercise. As a result, we tend to have lower self-esteem or self-worth and feel bad about ourselves.

I have, at times, used societal expectations as a motivator to stay in shape. I feel enormous pressure to "walk the walk" or "look the part" in terms of my physical appearance. What kind of person would I be to tell you that you should be lean and eat healthy foods, and then not be able to do it myself? I'd feel like a giant hypocrite, so it motivates me to take care of myself and make healthy decisions. This type of motivation is called *extrinsic motivation*—where your motivation comes from the external or surrounding environment.

Extrinsic motivators allow you to earn a reward or avoid some type of punishment, whether real or perceived. In my case, my "punishment" is that I feel that if I were overweight, I'd be chastised or looked down upon for not being able to be a role model. This may or may not be true.

Now, what would happen if my situation changed? Perhaps something happens that causes me to become depressed and gain some extra weight. Does that make me a failure? Maybe, maybe not. It would depend on who's judging me. This is why external motivators are good for getting people *started* on weight loss, but they lose their incentive fast.

Who doesn't want to be smart, beautiful, successful, and healthy? Pretty much every client I've worked with wants to have those qualities. The problem with that is that there is *always* someone skinnier than you are—someone smarter, someone prettier. People are also fickle. What's good enough today won't be good enough tomorrow. You'll have to do better, then. And sometimes, despite our best efforts, we fail to meet our health or fitness goals due to circumstances outside our control.

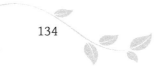

If we solely base our self-confidence on those superficial values, our self-esteem will be crushed the minute someone better than us comes along or we experience setbacks in life, which is going to happen, I promise. Extrinsic motivators only last so long, and then you need to rely on some other form of motivation to keep you going.

This is where *intrinsic motivation* comes in. Intrinsic motivators are the reasons that come from within yourself. They are personally rewarding and encourage you to keep pushing yourself even when the going gets tough. I do my best to eat healthy and work out regularly for a number of reasons. It isn't always easy. I don't always enjoy it. I just need to get it done. I make it a priority so that I have strong bones and muscles to prevent or reduce injuries in the future. I do it to reduce the chance of getting the diseases and medical conditions that run in my family. I do it to keep mentally healthy and balanced. But those are just *my* personal reasons. You need to find your own that motivate you.

Many of my clients start working out or eating healthier because I've encouraged them to do so or because they were told to by their doctors. They end up continuing with those healthy habits because they feel better, have more energy, and want to continue to feel that way.

I had been working with Ted for approximately six months. He either needed to have his diabetic medication increased or change his diet and activity level because his blood sugars were consistently too high. Ted was adamant that he was not going to start another medication, despite receiving the new prescription from his doctor. After several months of teaching Ted how to eat properly and encouraging him to walk, even for just five minutes a day, I got nowhere. Ted just wasn't ready to make changes.

Then one day, Ted went in to see the doctor and popped into my office after his appointment. He told me that he had started making changes to his diet and that it really wasn't that hard after all. He had even started walking and was up to ten minutes every day. He had lost a few pounds and was feeling much more energetic. Ted had to find his own reasons to make changes and start when *he* was ready, on *his own terms*.

When a person is already motivated by intrinsic factors, it's best not to introduce other incentives or extrinsic factors, as it may take away some of the drive or motivation to continue the activity. I've seen contests where participants can win prizes for regular attendance at the gym, fitness class, or yoga studio (external motivation). Initially, most people are motivated to go, and they enjoy winning prizes. However, once the contest is over, many of the people who were attending regularly start to dwindle and eventually stop coming. They are no longer getting prizes for attending workouts, and they lose their motivation.

Here are some examples of the difference between extrinsic and intrinsic motivators.

Extrinsic Motivators	Intrinsic Motivators
Trying new foods because your diet has them included as mandatory items	Trying new foods because you like experiencing new tastes
Exercising because someone is making you	Exercising because it makes you feel strong, energized, and mentally balanced
Meditating because you've read that it's good for you	Meditating regularly because it helps you think clearly and be more focused in your day
Losing weight to please someone else (doctor, partner)	Losing weight to decrease the pain in your hips, knees, and ankles
Quitting smoking because your work implemented a new no smoking policy	Quitting smoking because you want to be able to breathe better and not cough all the time

Now that you've got a better understanding of the different types of motivators, you can start to identify what motivates you. Take a few minutes to evaluate some of your own reasons for wanting to make lifestyle changes.

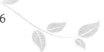

Extrinsic motivators (external reasons—earn a reward/avoid a punishment)

....

....

....

....

....

....

Intrinsic motivators (internal reasons—personally rewarding)

....

....

....

....

....

....

Great job! Now that you've got some different reasons that help give you motivation, it's time to start implementing changes. The next section will give you some tips and tricks for making healthy food choices.

Chapter Ten

Food Choices

W hen making food choices, I've noticed that people create their decisions based on three key criteria: convenience, cost, and health.

Most people generally want foods that are quick, easy to grab, and don't take a lot of time—if any—to prepare. That's convenience for you. It's an "I want it now" mentality. In terms of cost, I've never met a someone who willingly spent more on food just because they wanted to burn through more money. We all want to save money on food if we can. Some of us just pay more for it because we want the health benefits that come with increased cost. Which leads us to the nutritional benefits of our food. Not everything we put in our bodies is healthy. Some of us value the health of a certain food item more than the other aspects of choice.

Unfortunately, it's nearly impossible for us to have all three options at the same time. In fact, most times, we can only have two of the three choices, like a Euler diagram. This concept falls on the idea of the Theory of Constraints or the Iron Triangle, where we are limited in achieving our goals by a constraint, and it stipulates that there is *always* a constraint.

When making food choices, those constraints are cost, convenience, and health. You must consider, give up, or change one priority in order to get the other two top priorities.

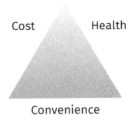

Cost   Health

Convenience

Let's look at the three different scenarios:

Cost and Convenience

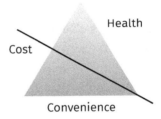

Health

Cost

Convenience

If we draw the line across the triangle, choosing cost and convenience, we often sacrifice the health benefits of the food. Options that are cheap and convenient tend to cause poor health outcomes. Foods that fall into this category are fast food, meals from poor-quality chain restaurants, everything in the snack aisle, and instant or frozen meals. It's also most cereals, pasta, breads, crackers, pop, and juice. Ideally, these foods should be eaten only occasionally, if ever. However, many people end up eating them simply because they can't afford to eat healthier foods.

Options for choosing healthier foods without sacrificing cost and convenience would be to buy bulk vegetables like bushels of carrots and potatoes or larger bags of plain rice, and cook them in bigger batches so less prep time is needed.

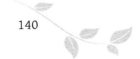

Convenience and Health

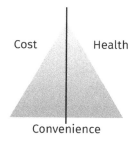

Foods that are convenient and healthy tend to cost more. These foods may be pre-chopped and packaged vegetables that you can easily turn into quick meals, or they may be vegetable platters or salads that are already prepared. To keep some dollars in your pocket and save on cost, work with friends or neighbors to batch-prepare healthy foods. This saves on cost and helps get the job of chopping and other prep work done much faster.

Health and Cost

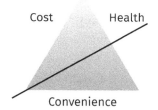

Foods that are healthy and cheap generally take more time to prepare or produce, meaning they aren't as convenient. Growing your own garden would be a prime example of these kinds of foods. It requires a large time investment but a much smaller financial investment. Getting produce from a community supported agriculture program (CSA) or from a farmers' market is a more convenient way to get healthy and inexpensive food.

Which Option is Best?

Overall, you have to decide where your priorities lie. You can't have your cake and eat it too! It's important to decide what's most important or which factor absolutely can't change.

The biggest holdup for people seems to be tied to finances. That being said, you can choose between food that's healthy or food that's convenient, likely not both. If you value optimal health, you have to be prepared to put in a bit of time and elbow grease to eat healthy. The consequence of eating convenient food is that it's often not optimal quality, and it's lacking in health priorities. This is where you can weigh the pros and cons and ultimately make the decision that best resonates with your values.

Nutrition Optimization

To wrap up the Nutrition section, here's a four-step strategy to help clean up your diet and get you on the road to eating healthier.

1) Clean up

Clean up your house, empty out your cupboards, and throw out the junk food you've been hiding. Even that secret stash hiding you-know-where! Remove processed foods and foods that contain sugar and excess salt. Look at labels on foods, sauces, condiments, cookies, crackers, pasta, etc., and get rid of anything that has ingredients that you don't know what they are or what they do.

Many people suggest not to eat anything you can't pronounce. Inspired by that movement, food producers have changed the names of ingredients so that they are easier to pronounce. In other words, just because you can pronounce it doesn't mean you should eat it. You may be able to say MSG, xanthan gum, or corn syrup, but it doesn't mean they are healthful for you to be eating regularly.

When doing a house clean-out, there are two ways to go about it: all at once or gradually, over time. Some people need the "rip off the band-aid"

approach, where they throw everything away all at once. Some people hate throwing food away and need to change gradually over time. Either way, it has to get done. Clean out your house, and take no longer than one month to do it. This will help you avoid temptation, and it will prevent you from falling back into old habits.

I'm not very good at moderating food and only having a little bit. I will eat while I'm baking if it's available or hidden in the basement freezer—so I don't bake very often or keep those items around the house to tempt me. Out of sight, out of mind! You can apply a similar method as outlined in Marie Kondo's *The Life-Changing Magic of Tidying Up*. Ask yourself if each piece of food will bring you greater health and nourish your body. If not, it's time to get rid of it and not buy it again. This same approach should go for your pets' food and treats too. If junk food isn't healthy for you, it sure isn't for Fido either!

2) Stock up

Once you have cleaned out the house, you will likely find that your cupboards are quite empty, and you will need more food options to choose from. Stock up on healthy food so that you have lots of nutritious foods to eat when you are hungry. When you open the refrigerator door or the cupboards looking for something to eat, the foods that stare back are essentially being marketed to you. By marketing healthy food choices, you will have more willpower to make healthy choices. You also have more of a moral obligation to eat the food in front of you, since you've already spent money on it. It's more work to leave the house to go get junk food, which helps cut down on impulse eating.

When I went through the transition to getting rid of most processed foods in my home, I was completely shocked at how bare my cupboards were. I wasn't sure what I would eat because there was no food in the house. Over time, I learned many ways to prepare vegetables quickly and easily, and I filled my fridge and freezer with many different foods that I hadn't eaten before. The cupboards and pantry filled in again, this time with more spices than I ever thought possible. I've currently got over fifty different varieties and am still adding more! My pantry has been filled with cooking appliances and other utensils that make food preparation much easier.

3) Experiment

Try lots of new foods and new cooking techniques. Try new recipes and develop new healthy habits. Track your food intake in a food journal to identify how you feel with different types of foods and modify as needed. Journaling will help you separate what you *think* you are eating from what you are *actually* eating.

It's also important to give your body time to adapt to a new diet before writing it off as one that doesn't work for you. Take one to three months on a set diet to allow your body time to adjust to the changes. This will help you identify what types of foods help you feel most energetic and what foods sap your mental willpower and energy, so that you can learn to make your own healthy food choices.

4) Optimize

This is where you may want to consult with a health care professional to identify ideal macro and micronutrient ratios for yourself. You should stick to ratios of macronutrients (protein, carbohydrate, fat) where you look the best, feel the best, and also have a good blood profile. Remember that your body will change over time, so you may need to adjust the ratios as your stress levels or sleep patterns change and as you get older. What works for you at age forty may no longer work for you at age fifty.

Pillar 3: Exercise

"Take care of your body. It's the only place you have
to live."

—Jim Rohn

"If I don't feel confident about my body, I'm not going
to sit at home and feel sorry for myself and not do
something about it. It's all about taking action and not
being lazy. So you do the work, whether it's fitness or
whatever. It's about getting up, motivating yourself and
just doing it."

—Kim Kardashian

"If a man achieves victory over his body, who in the
world can exercise power over him? He who rules
himself rules over the whole world."

—Vinoba Bhave

Chapter Eleven

What is Exercise?

*L*et's start by clarifying the difference between exercise and activity. There are some days that I literally want to rip my hair out because of what people count as "exercise." Walter works from home and would go up and down the stairs three times in the day, counting that as his exercise. He also thought that walking at the grocery store and shoveling his four-foot-long sidewalk once a week was exercise. I couldn't convince him otherwise.

These things are not exercises. They are activities. Call it movement. Call it activity. Call it whatever you like. It's not exercise!

Activity

Activity is any physical movement of the body that uses up energy. Most people count their activities of daily living (ADL) as exercise. These ADLs are the things you need to do in the day, like cooking, laundry, housework, or yard work, and often involve going up and down the stairs a few times in the day. These activities are movements that you perform in your day. General activity can also include taking the stairs instead of the elevator or parking at the back of the parking lot so that you have to walk further.

Marina is a nurse on a busy unit. She works twelve-hour shifts and is up and down the unit all day. Her job is very physical, and she's often turning patients or helping transfer them in and out of bed. Despite being very active in her job, Marina is overweight and can't seem to lose the unwanted pounds. The problem is that her body has already adapted to that current level of activity, and she is no longer getting additional benefit from it. In order to see further improvements in her health, Marina will either need to do more activity, exercise, or address the other pillars of her health.

Some people get out of breath from performing activities (e.g., walking up stairs) but in most cases, that comes from being deconditioned or out of shape rather than it being a difficult task. While I believe that we should all work to keep our activity level higher, we don't get the same health benefits from activity as we do from exercise.

Activity should be performed on a daily basis to keep active and reduce the loss of function. Too often, I see this in seniors who stop being active. Their bodies just waste away. Keep your body moving; it's truly a case of *use it or lose it.*

Be as active as your situation allows you to be. Maybe you just had surgery and need to take some time to recover at home. Working out might just push you over the edge and make your recovery take longer. Start introducing activity into your day gradually as you tolerate it. Overall, I encourage you to try to be active in some way every day. Activity is a good thing.

Exercise

Exercise is activity that is planned, structured, and repeatable. The goal of exercise is to maintain or increase your current level of fitness. It's also to prevent the natural declines that happen with age. From the ripe old age of *thirty*, it's all downhill. Okay, perhaps I'm being a bit dramatic! We do, however, have a natural decline in muscle mass and bone mass starting around age thirty. This decline starts out slowly and increases as we get

older, generally accelerating around fifty years of age. The rate of decline is slightly different for everyone and usually happens earlier for women than men due to the hormonal changes during menopause. This decline in muscle mass and bone density can largely be reduced or prevented by engaging in exercise that helps to maintain strength as we age.

Unlike activity, exercise gets your heart rate up for longer periods of time and gives the added benefit of building muscle mass and/or bone density. Exercise also helps you maintain better posture, alignment, or ergonomics, allowing you to move your body as it was intended to move rather than coming up with awkward movement compensations that often lead to injury.

Exercise is done over and over again to provide a repeatable stressor on the body, which in turn leads to a strengthening of the system. If you only walk up and down your stairs six times in the day (activity), it may be spaced too far apart to get the desired benefit. Some activities push into the exercise category, such as digging a trench in your yard, shoveling gravel, or moving a load of heavy boxes. These activities involve moving a load repeatedly for an extended time.

I'd also like to draw some special attention to rehabilitation from an injury or illness. Activity or exercise that's done when someone is healthy is completely different from when they are recovering and trying to rehabilitate after a period of weakness or immobility. Activities that used to be mundane or easy may become intense exercises after an injury. This book does not specifically address rehabilitation, as that's a whole other ball game and could be an entire book on its own. In some conditions like lupus or multiple sclerosis, there is a delicate balance between exercising to build or maintain strength and overdoing things. Use discretion when participating in exercise programs, and make sure you get a balance of rest to receive the benefit from all your hard work.

Fitness

It's one thing to exercise, it's another thing to achieve different levels of fitness.

Merriam-Webster's Dictionary:

fitness

1: the quality or state of being fit

2: the capacity of an organism to survive and transmit its genotype to reproductive offspring as compared to competing organisms; *also*: the contribution of an allele or genotype to the gene pool of subsequent generations as compared to that of other alleles or genotypes

Here's what I like about the dictionary—the first definition is simple and to the point, yet still does not clarify what "fit" means. Although the second definition seems to focus on biology too much, I believe there is some validity to the definition. If you are unable to either physically engage in the act of sex due to being obese or are unable to conceive due to a vast array of health conditions, you are of poor fitness. (While I recognize that there are genetic causes of infertility, several common cases of infertility can be remedied by improving the fitness of both partners.)

Similar to the Merriam-Webster's Dictionary, Wikipedia mentions the genetic components of fitness and also looks at various components of sports and fitness, including health. This raises the point that you can be fit but not necessarily healthy. This is especially true when we look at most bodybuilders or high-level athletes who are pushing the boundaries of fitness.

For the purposes of this book, when I refer to fitness, it means that you are fit enough to accomplish *more* than your routine daily tasks with sufficient energy to respond to an unexpected event, and that you possess a balance of cardiovascular health, agility, flexibility, muscular strength, endurance, power, balance, and body composition.

What's the Point of Exercise?

Now that you have a better understanding of what exercise is, you're probably wondering why you should even consider doing it. Especially if you hate exercising!

There are so many benefits of exercise that you'd get bored reading them all. Here are some of my favorite benefits:

- Blood sugar and blood pressure regulation
- Increased HDL (that's the good, protective cholesterol)
- Decreased fat mass (Who wants extra fat? No one—let's kick it to the curb!)
- Increased muscle mass, joint stability
- Improved balance and coordination
- Improved posture
- Increase metabolism (so you can burn more energy just sitting around)
- Improved self-esteem, self-confidence, positive energy, body image
- Improved focus and concentration, social involvement/engagement
- Reduction in sick/injury time at work
- Improved quality of life
- Reduction in stress/anxiety/depression
- Can be as effective as antidepressants (without the side effects of weight gain)
- Reduced injuries
- Improved immune system
- Reduction in type two diabetes, obesity, cardiovascular disease

Wow! That's a lot of benefits from one small lifestyle strategy. It's almost hard to understand why everyone doesn't exercise. However, before you start to exercise, you'll want to check with your doctor to make sure that it's safe for you to do so. A common health screening form is called the PARmed-X, which identifies common risk factors that may prevent you from being active. It screens for pregnancy, cardiovascular disease, infections, or metabolic conditions that prevent or limit you from participating in certain exercises.

For people who fall into the *absolute contraindications* category, it is recommended not to exercise because the risk of injury or death may be too high. That being said, I highly recommend talking to your doctor to identify if *all* exercise is off the table or if you are still safe to perform gentle balance exercises, stretching, or reduced resistance training using elastic bands, as these activities often have little cardiovascular impact.

Again, focus on what you can do, not what you can't. For those few people who have been told that any type of exercise is too risky, it will be especially important for you to balance your other pillars of health in order to stay well.

What's Your Starting Point?

Rather than getting hung up on where you *used to* be or where you *want to* be, the best place to start is exactly where you are right now. The past is the past, and the future hasn't happened yet, so accept that your fitness is currently what it is because of what you did or didn't do. Own it! And then set a plan for moving forward. I don't care if you used to play varsity football or were in ballet. What are you doing right now? That's what matters. Read through the following descriptions to determine what kind of athlete you are because we are all athletes when we move our bodies as they are meant to be.

Beginner

You are just starting out for the first time ever, or perhaps you haven't started training consistently. You may be healthy (or not) but generally don't have a strong athletic background. Perhaps you used to work out regularly, but it's been a long time since you worked out. If it has been a while, you will likely move through this phase quicker than if you've never worked out before.

Goals of training:

- **Improve your neuromuscular efficiency**

  Say what? *Neuro* is your nerve, *muscular* is your muscles. This part of training is trying to get your nerves and muscles on the same page so they work together as a team. Your goal is to create a nerve conduction superhighway, but in the beginning, it will be more like driving off-road through a bumpy field (more on this later). This is the biggest adaptation that most people experience when they start weight training, which explains why you get such a quick increase in strength right away. These gains level off once neuromuscular efficiency is achieved in an exercise. Your future gains will come more from increased muscle mass, which occurs more slowly.

- **Motor control**

Move in a slow and controlled manner through the entire range of motion so that your muscles can work in their lengthened position and give the appropriate feedback to your brain.

- **Anatomical adaptation**

This is where your tissues adapt to the movement you are perform- ing. Your muscles, tendons, and ligaments get stronger after you exercise, making your joints more stable and able to tolerate force.

- **Controlled range of motion**

During your exercises, work through your full range of motion as long as you are able to control the movement. If you try a pull-up and end up dropping down fast because you can't lower yourself slowly, you're putting yourself at risk for injury. Either hold off on these types of exercises until you can control the entire range of motion, or decrease the range of motion you work in.

Intermediate

Move on to the intermediate level of training once you have developed a level of general fitness. You'll be able to do most basic movements with good technique and will have the ability to maintain some intensity for a longer period of time. At this point, you'll have better body awareness and will know what your body parts are doing at the same time.

Goals of training:

- **Increased movement, complexity, and force**

As you build your neuromuscular pathways, you'll be able to in- crease the complexity of your movements and do more variations of the same movement pattern. You'll also be able to generate more force in the same movement patterns that you are used to doing.

- **Increased range of motion**

  As I mentioned in the pull-up example for the beginner athlete, you'll now be able to increase that range of motion with strength throughout the entire range. This prevents you from being limited in movement choices by your lack of strength.

- **Decreased reaction time**

  Now that you know how to move, you'll be able to start integrating reaction time into movements, doing more agility exercises or unpredictable movements that keep your mind and body guessing what's coming next. When working on decreasing reaction time, you'll likely make many mistakes, but that will improve with practice.

Advanced

This stage of training may not be for everyone. Here, you'll be able to sustain exercise for prolonged periods of time or exert maximal force. Movements are easy now, but you're working on generating more force or power through the movement. Typically, individuals in advanced levels of training are in some type of competition that drives them to increase their performance, but they don't necessarily need to be elite-level athletes.

Goals of training:

- **Faster movement**

  You've mastered the movement at slow and controlled speeds. Now, it's time to kick it up into high gear. Start training with faster movements for an added challenge.

- **Dynamic ability**

  You can now do full range of movement exercises using a variety of speeds and weights. You can break down the exercise into smaller

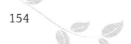

segments to improve one specific part of a larger movement or do the exercise in slow motion to see where it may be breaking down.

- **High movement complexity, high force movements**

  You've now mastered that neuromuscular complex and are taking it to the extreme. Your exercises are complex, using multiple planes of movement, uneven surfaces, and under less than ideal circumstances using a load.

- **Reactive movement patterns**

  You'll also be able to respond to uncertain circumstances faster with less conscious thought.

This gives you a better idea of where you stand in your current fitness level. You might be really clear about where you sit, or perhaps you think that you cross over into different levels of athletic ability. It is possible to be a beginner in one movement and advanced in another, so don't get too hung up on where you start. You can cross between these zones, going back and forth, depending on what exercise you are doing, the highest level you've previously achieved, and where you're starting from.

Chapter Twelve

Components of Exercise and Fitness

*Y*ou now understand all the amazing benefits of exercising and you know where to start, but you may not be sure what you should be doing. There are lots of different types of exercise programs out there, such as fitness classes, weight training, swimming, biking running, yoga, and Pilates. New types of exercises and new fads are coming out all the time. What they all have in common is that they target components of fitness, giving you benefits specific to that exercise. Let's explore the different components of fitness to give you a better understanding.

Cardiovascular

Cardiovascular fitness, also called cardio, is the heart's ability to deliver blood to working muscles and their ability to use it. As you gain cardiovascular fitness, you'll be able to work harder or faster with less effort. Some examples of cardiovascular fitness include walking, running, hiking, swimming and biking. Now list three activities that you'd like to try to boost your cardiovascular fitness:

Flexibility

Flexibility refers to the ability to achieve range of motion around a joint without being impeded by excess tissue such as too much fat or muscle. You don't want to be flexible just for the sake of being flexible; however, you do want to be able to move without limitation during your chosen activity. A few examples of flexibility include stretching, yoga, Pilates, or simply touching your toes. Now list three activities that you'd like to try to boost your flexibility:

Muscular Strength

Muscular strength is the extent to which muscles can maximally exert force. A few examples of muscular strength include performing a heavy or maximal weight deadlift, squat, or bench press. The maximum weight you can lift will be relative to where your current fitness is and how well your nervous system works.

If you are just starting out, you'll want to go easy on this type of exercise so that you don't end up injured. Strength exercises are done in lower repetitions, usually somewhere between one to five repetitions in an exercise set. Now list three exercises that you'd like to try to boost your muscular strength:

Muscular Endurance

Muscular endurance is the extent to which your muscles can repeatedly exert a force. This refers to how many times you can do a movement over and over again before the muscle fatigues and you need to stop. Endurance exercises are typically weight-training exercises done in sets of repetitions. Endurance exercises are done in higher repetitions, usually ranging from eight to twenty repetitions in an exercise set.

Endurance training often brings up thoughts of distance events such as marathons, triathlons, or long distance swimming and cycling events.

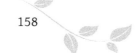

These also use muscular endurance, as your muscles need to repeat a movement over and over again. Now list three exercises that you'd like to try to boost your muscular endurance:

....

Power

Power refers to the ability to exert maximum muscular contraction instantly in an explosive burst of movements. The two components of power are strength and speed. In order to improve power output, you'll need to increase your muscular strength or speed up the timing of the movement. Power activities are generally not used for beginner athletes due to the need to have solid biomechanics to avoid injury.

That's not to say that they can't be done. You'll just want to make sure you do them in a controlled manner with a coach to ensure good technique. Some examples of power exercises are jumping, plyometrics, or a sprint start in a race. Now list three activities that you'd like to try to boost your power:

....

Agility

Agility is the ability to perform a series of repetitive, explosive power movements in opposing directions. To perform agility movements well, you need to have a good foundation of power, muscular strength, and some muscular endurance. A few examples of agility include running zig-zag patterns, following ladder drills, or quick changes of direction. That being said, agility can start very simple too.

Imagine you've just recovered from a leg injury. Your agility might look more like walking down the sidewalk and avoiding the rock in line with your trajectory. Or stepping to the side to avoid getting run over by the toddler on his tricycle. While these movements aren't extreme agility, we do need to be able to respond to uneven or unpredictable terrain, which agility helps us do. Now list three activities that you'd like to try to boost your agility:

....

Balance

Balance is the ability to control the body's position, either stationary (standing on one foot) or while moving (one leg squat). Some other examples of balance include standing on one foot when you put your socks on, using wobble boards, or standing on uneven surfaces. Balance is definitely an area that more people need to work on and is often neglected. It involves an interaction of input from your visual (eyes), proprioceptive (feeling/touch), and vestibular (inner ear) systems. To promote or maintain balance, it's important to work on all three of these components.

A simple progression of balance is to start by standing on one foot. This works the proprioceptive system, as the foot and leg muscles respond to the swaying or body movement, they adjust to keep you upright. Once standing on a foot is no longer a challenge, do the same exercise looking at the ceiling. That changes the position of the vestibular system, making your inner ear tell your body something totally different than what your eyes and feet are telling you, ultimately making the exercise more challenging. If that's still too easy for you, close your eyes! That knocks out the visual feedback, taking the difficulty up a notch. You can follow this same progression to make any balance exercise more challenging. Now list three things that you'd like to try to boost your balance:

....

Body Composition

This refers to the amounts of body fat and lean body tissue found on your body. Your body composition is affected by factors such as genetics, diet, exercise, metabolism, stress level, hormonal balance, and sleep. It's often not just one of these factors that cause body composition to go

up or down, but rather a complex interaction between all of them. Body composition is often measured by a body mass index scale (BMI), which I'm sure you've heard of by now.

I have a love-hate relationship with the BMI scale in that it's good for some things but not for others. Remember: The BMI scale is only a tool to measure body composition and does not give the whole picture. It accounts for the difference between your height and weight without accounting for what your weight is made up of. Your body weight comes from your bone density, muscle mass, fat mass, water, and everything else that makes up your organs, blood vessels, hair, and skin. Some of those variables will change very little (like your bones), while muscle mass and fat mass can change dramatically during your lifetime.

I've worked with athletes who have three percent body fat and are considered obese on the BMI scale because of their large ratio of muscle mass. On the flip side, I've worked with "skinny-fat" clients who have a normal BMI but have too much fat and not enough muscle on their frame.

Recognize that the BMI scale is not perfect but can be useful for tracking changes in body composition. Most average people do well with using the BMI scale to get an idea of their risk of developing health problems. The higher your BMI, the higher your risk of getting preventable chronic diseases.

Rather than comparing yourself to other people and justifying your own weight, start comparing yourself to yourself. Track what your BMI is from year to year, with the goal of preventing an increase in BMI with increased fat mass. If you are adding muscle mass through exercise and your BMI goes up, this increase is not associated with the same health risks as gaining fat.

The FITT Formula

The FITT formula is a way to help you adjust and manipulate exercise to ensure a continued benefit from it over time. It stands for Frequency,

Intensity, Time, and Type. I'll go through each of those variables to help you learn how to adjust your own exercise program so that you are able to continue to benefit from it without needing to hire a personal trainer or coach to give you support. (Although I highly encourage having a coach or personal trainer, I fully realize that this is not financially feasible for many people. It's also not always necessary if you are doing simple exercises at home or a walking program.)

Exercise can be adjusted based on the intensity of the activity and according to your fitness goals.

Frequency

This is how often you are doing an exercise—how many days or times per week you exercise. Your frequency may vary from once every month all the way up to several times per day, depending on what type of activity you are doing. To achieve continued benefit, you'll want to attain a balance between overdoing it and not doing it often enough.

Lower-intensity exercises or stretches can potentially be performed more often than higher-intensity exercises. For example, you are able to perform postural exercises daily, as these muscles are designed for endurance, whereas if you were doing a maximum weight power clean, you'd want to do it less often to ensure appropriate recovery.

Intensity

Intensity refers to how hard the exercise is or how much effort goes into it. Some exercises will have much more potential for variability than others. For example, you can only stretch *so hard* or *so intense*. Ever hear of the stretch Olympics, where the best stretcher wins? It just wouldn't happen. A squat has a much higher range for intensity. Someone doing rehabilitation after surgery might start with a partial squat and then progress to a full-range bodyweight squat as they get stronger. Others might perform a weighted squat or add a jump for maximal intensity. There is a very broad range in exercise intensity.

Intensity can be changed by the speed of your movement. This pace is called your tempo. If you are doing a much slower movement tempo, it

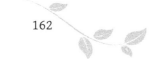

will increase the length of time the load is applied to each muscle, which makes the muscle work harder to stabilize, in turn, increasing the intensity. Faster tempos are much more demanding but need to be eased into so as to ensure that correct biomechanical techniques are used.

You can also vary the joint's range of motion. The greater the range of motion, the more intense the exercise will be; in contrast, the smaller the range of motion, the less intense the exercise will be. It's hard to do a really intense exercise through a tiny range of motion—these smaller movements are usually meant to target the weakest part of the movement. To adjust the intensity of walking, you could progressively increase your speed to get added benefit. That same old pace you've always done will eventually stop giving you new benefits.

Another way to alter the intensity is to adjust the complexity of the movement. A toe tap would be a much less intense exercise than a pull-up because it's using a much smaller muscle groups. The pull-up recruits much more muscle fibers and expends much greater energy.

Time

This is how long you are doing the exercise. Exercise time can be increased or decreased to adjust the effectiveness of the workout, but time can only be increased to a certain point before the duration is unsustainable. You've only got so many hours in the day and can only fit so much into your day. If every few weeks you had to walk for a longer time to keep getting benefit from it, at some point you'd eventually run out of enough hours in the day to get other things done. This makes time a limiting factor for most people.

Time is also used as an excuse for why you can't workout. You might think, "*I'm too busy to exercise.*" This makes it a difficult variable to adjust—and just as difficult as some of the other variables. Time is also not necessarily an isolated indicator of how beneficial your workout is. Some of my clients have done really great workouts in only twenty minutes. Others have gone on an hour-long walk but only covered one kilometer— much less effective.

Type

This refers to the actual exercise you are doing. There is a huge variety of types of exercises. You've probably heard that "variety is the spice of life"—and that's quite true when it comes to exercise, especially if you want to be well-rounded. Not to be confused with trying to be round. That's not the direction I want to move you in! You'll find some movements that you don't like or don't want to do as often as other exercises. Do your best to find exercises that you enjoy doing so that you are more likely to stick with them and so that you can target different aspects of fitness that you are lacking. With fitness, you want to be well rounded, so you'll want to work on symmetry between body parts and the different components of fitness.

For example, if you are training to be a better sprinter, speed and power are going to be much more important to your fitness routine than endurance. However, that's not to say that you should ignore all endurance activities. It would just be a smaller component of your program. The higher level of athlete you are, the more specific your fitness routine will likely be. But for most of us, if we do a little bit of everything, we'll come out on top. This will help prevent injuries and boredom and will keep your body much more balanced.

Manipulating the FITT Formula

When you are looking to make changes in your current fitness program, start by evaluating what you are doing and look at the different variables that are available to change.

Walking is a common exercise, so I'll use that as an example. If you have been walking for ten minutes once per week as your initial activity, how could you manipulate your walks to get more benefit from them? You could increase your total time by adding an extra minute, or you could increase the intensity by walking faster for those same ten minutes. To vary the frequency, you would walk for ten minutes two to three times per week. If you *only* want to walk for exercise, you could vary the type by walking on different terrain: going up and down stairs, taking uneven

dirt paths, or going up and down hills to get more benefit than you would by just walking on flat pathways.

Principles of Exercise

Progression

In order to achieve a training effect, exercise intensity or duration must gradually increase over time. These variables should be adjusted somewhere around every four to six weeks to continue to benefit the body. They should be increased by no more than a 10 percent total adjustment between all variables to prevent injury or overtraining. That means that you are only going to adjust one of these variables at a time, not all of them at once.

The reason you don't want to adjust more than 10 percent at a time is to give the connective tissues (ligaments, tendons) in your body time to adapt to the progressive overload without tearing or getting inflamed or injured. The principle of progression should also be applied to the FITT formula so that you aren't manipulating all the variables at one time, which can lead to changes that are too great for the body to adapt to. Pick only one aspect of the FITT formula to change at a time!

Specificity

To achieve a training benefit, the type of exercise done must be related to the desired effect. As an example, to improve cardiovascular fitness, you must do activities that get your heart rate up. Makes sense, right? You wouldn't do ballet to get better at doing pull-ups.

Nadine was doing lots of walking and wondered why she wasn't losing weight. She was past menopause and felt that her diet, sleep, and stress level were all in balance. Her scenario is all too common. Middle-aged menopausal women undergo a hormonal shift that often results in weight gain. While this story is common, it doesn't *have* to happen—at least not to the extent that it usually does.

165

Although walking is a fantastic exercise and provides many benefits, it's typically not specific enough to help prevent excess weight gain in menopausal women. In these cases, many women see a benefit from doing weight training to boost their muscle mass and keep their metabolism higher at rest.

Recuperation

In order to achieve a training effect, there must be an appropriate rest or recovery time from the exercise to promote adaptation of muscle, tendon, and ligament tissues. Appropriate rest can be achieved by alternating the type of training or the body part being trained. In weight training, a common routine is to do upper body training one day and lower body the next day instead of doing total body workouts every day.

Rest is equally important as exercise. If you work out too hard without giving your body adequate rest, you'll never heal or get stronger, which is what you are trying to accomplish by working out. On the flip side, you don't want to train too infrequently with extended gaps of rest because you won't be pushing your body enough to receive the benefits. If you lift weights only one or two times per month, it probably isn't often enough to gain a progression in your strength.

The more intense the exercise, the more rest you need between workouts. Less intense exercises can be performed more often. Postural exercises can be performed daily, as these muscles are designed to work all the time, while other larger muscle groups need more rest to reap the benefit.

Overload/Overtraining

This principle is tied to the concept of rest, or rather, the lack of rest. Failure to get enough rest and recovery time between workouts may lead to injuries or chronically feeling fatigued.

You can't expect to get fit by sitting on your stationary bike; you actually have to pedal it! The idea of "overload" means that you need to provide a load to your muscles to get a benefit. As you get fitter, you'll need to keep overloading your system to continue to get that same benefit.

If taken too far, however, overload can result in overtraining, which results in a decrease in the benefit from exercise. Tamara, a high-drive triathlete, always felt that she had to do *more*. She always did more than I asked her to do. When creating her workout routine, I eventually started scheduling *half* of what I actually wanted her to run because I knew she'd do more. This all-or-nothing mentality often leads to overtraining and prevents athletes from hitting their goals because they burn out or get injured before their goal event.

Key Takeaways

In order to get continuous benefit from your exercises, make sure you keep progressing what you are doing. Do exercises that are specific to the area that you are trying to improve. Make sure that you get the right balance of rest and work so that you are able to get the maximum benefit from your workout. It's always best to find activities that you are naturally talented at and enjoy doing, as you'll be more likely to stick to them.

Chapter Thirteen

Deepening Your Knowledge

T hat was a whole lot of theory I just threw at you! So what does it all mean and how do you start to pull it together so you can use it? Now that you understand a bit about how exercise programs are put together, it's time to start applying those principles.

Slow to fast

Ever jump into an activity that you used to do and end up injured after a few weeks? Or perhaps you've seen someone do an exercise in the gym, and you just started to do it on your own because it looked cool. You'll find that it takes time to learn how to perform a movement correctly. By starting a new exercise in a slow and controlled manner, you are allowing your nervous system to adapt to the movement pattern. Your goal isn't just to improve muscle strength; your goal is to improve nerve conduction.

The first few times you do a movement, it's like driving off-road through a field. It's bumpy, shaky, and sometimes you end up off course. With repetition of perfect technique, you build up the memory of where your body needs to move. That improvement in nerve conduction turns the bumpy path in the field into a gravel road, then a paved road, and eventually, a superhighway as you get better at the technique. Practice truly makes perfect.

Go slow to go fast, and reinforce perfect technique. The details matter when you start. You'll reduce the risk of injury and will have better results in the long run.

Stable to unstable

Start from a foundation that is incredibly stable before you progress to unstable surfaces. The focus over the last ten years in the fitness industry has been to use unstable objects such as wobble boards or exercise balls while doing other exercises. Greg liked to combine complex exercises to get greater benefits. He used to stand with a wobble board under each foot while doing complex upper body cable exercises. His form was horrible, and he came close to falling numerous times, often getting twisted in the cables. It was painful to watch, and no matter how much I suggested that this wasn't a safe exercise for Greg at the time, he refused to give up on it.

By starting a new exercise with a broad base of support (feet shoulder-width apart), you'll be able to reinforce good technique and adapt to the exercise. As you get better, you'll be able to shrink your base of support (feet closer together) and then progress to uneven surfaces. Had Greg started with just the upper body exercises, then done the balance exercises, then combined them, he would have been much more successful at doing them together.

Start with a nice, wide base of support, shrink your base, and then start adding other variables to make it more unstable. Other ways to move to unstable surfaces are to do exercises on different grades. Rather than walking on a flat path, walk up a hill, down a hill, or on a path pitched to one side. All these different angles make your body work in different ways, all with added benefits. Keep mixing it up! You can also use different surfaces to get different results. Walk on soft sand or hard-packed sand. Walk on cement and long grass. They all offer different benefits.

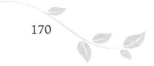

Known to unknown

The "known" are your very predictable exercises, where you know exactly what's going to happen. An example of a known exercise would be walking on a treadmill with the speed and incline set at one level. You know what's coming, and nothing changes until you hit stop. It's predictable.

To progress that to the unknown, you could put the treadmill on a variable program where it changes speed and incline on you randomly. You are forced to adapt to the changes it makes. Or you could go walk outside on a new trail in the mountains. You never know what's around the corner. Sometimes, the trail is straight up, while other times, it's slanted to the side.

Other examples of unknown training are working with a partner or trainer who gives you commands to perform. They could tell you to jump onto your right foot, then your left through a grid pattern on the floor—this activity is always changing and much more challenging.

Begin with exercise patterns that are known *before* jumping into unknown or uncontrolled situations that are beyond your skill level.

Low force to high force

This one makes a ton of sense for injury prevention. Force, in the context of exercise, refers to change of direction, lever length, and speed. Think of swinging a golf club, for example. The swing of the club uses rotation, a long lever arm, and high speed. Start with learning the basic body positioning to perform the movement correctly. Once you understand the basic movement, you can start to progress to a faster speed. You'll need to swing the club at a decent speed to get the feel for it so that you can perfect your technique, but you don't want to start by swinging the club as fast as possible.

Simple to complex

Earlier, we discussed the "field to superhighway" nerve analogy. Skipping simple movements and starting with complex movements would be like jumping onto a superhighway with training wheels on your bike. It just won't end well! Begin with basic movement patterns like a shoulder press or bicep curl before you start linking them together.

Pulling it together

You can now separate different movement patterns, and you know how to start simple, then progress to more challenging exercises. The next section will link the steps you need to do as you progress on your own exercise routine.

Periodization

"Periodization." Now that's a big, fancy word! In the fitness world, it's quite a common term, but most people I know have never heard of it before. Periodization refers to the cyclical nature of training in order to maximize your gains. Just as suggested by the principle of overtraining, if you work hard all the time, your body will eventually tire and be unable to perform at that same level.

What periodization does is take your workouts and break them up into different cycles or blocks to balance out the year. Some people refer to these blocks as pre-season, in-season, post-season, and off-season. Unless you're training for specific events, those terms mean nothing. However, that doesn't mean that you can't use those same principles to get fitter in everyday life. The other way to think about periodization is to go with the natural cycles that your body needs and craves, often in sync with the change of the seasons.

A full year would be considered your *macro-cycle*—the big cycle of your fitness plan. This is where you'll consider your long-term goals. What do you want to accomplish in the next year? If you are starting as a sedentary person, your broad plan might be to work out regularly so that you are able to lose forty pounds over the year. For most people, the broad focus of your training plan should be to build a large base of cardiovascular fitness and muscular fitness prior to focusing on strength, agility, and power.

The next stages of planning are your *meso-cycles* or medium-sized cycles that focus on the same adaptation in your training. You could choose to focus on aerobic training or building power in different meso-cycles. These cycles generally last between two to six weeks. Remember how we learned

that your body needs to change things up about every six weeks, to keep getting benefits from what you are doing? This cycle reinforces that!

The smallest cycle type is the *micro-cycle*, which is generally one week in length. They combine to make up the meso-cycle and typically build in intensity for a period of time, followed by a rest week with less or no activity.

Step One: What level of fitness are you?

(Beginner, Intermediate, Advanced)

Step Two: What phase of training are you in?

(Macro-cycle, Meso-cycle, Micro-cycle)

Step Three: What component of fitness do you want to focus on?

(Cardiovascular, Flexibility, Muscular Strength, Muscular Endurance, Power, Agility, Balance)

Step Four: Where are you currently in exercise progression?

(Slow/Fast, Stable/Unstable, Known/Unknown, Low/High, Simple/Complex)

Step Five: Which FITT Principle are you going to change?

(Frequency, Intensity, Time, Type)

Step Six: Which Fitness Principle are you going to apply?

(Progression, Specificity, Recuperation, Overload/Overtraining)

I'll now show you how to go through this process with walking as an example. I recommend walking as the first exercise for most people to start with when they are becoming active.

Step One: What level of fitness are you?

Beginner

Step Two: What phase of training are you in?

Macro-cycle: goal to walk 5 km
Meso-cycle: Increase walking by 0.5 km/month
Micro-cycle: walk 5 minutes once per week

Step Three: What component of fitness do you want to focus on?

Cardiovascular and Muscular Endurance

Step Four: Where are you currently in exercise progression?

Slow, Stable, Known, Low, Simple

Step Five: Which FITT Principle are you going to change?

Frequency: start with walking on a treadmill one time per week, progress to walking five times.

Time: once at five times per week, work on increasing time by no more than 10 percent each week, with the goal of walking for 30 minutes at a time.

Step Six: Which Fitness Principle are you going to apply?

Progression: gradual progression of walking

Specificity: walking specifically targets cardiovascular fitness and will help with goal of weight loss

Recuperation: low intensity with adequate recuperation time between walking sessions

Overload/Overtraining: once initial ramp-up phase is complete, walking increases by no more than 10 percent per week, in line with recommendations

You can now take this same formula and look at your current routine to determine what exercise you are doing, and you now have many ways that you can change the exercise to get continuous benefit from it.

What's a Good Exercise for Me?

By now, you're probably starting to feel more confident in creating your own exercise routine but still aren't quite sure what exercises you should be doing. Should you focus on cardio? Or maybe weights? You've heard yoga is good for you but don't love it. There are so many options to choose from. Here are some of the best questions to ask yourself to determine if an exercise is appropriate for you.

What is your goal?

Cathy's goal was to be really strong, lean, competitive in her age group in an Ironman, and to compete in three mountain bike races all in one year. On top of that, she's a mom, works a busy full-time job, and sits on a few

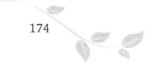

boards. While Cathy has amazingly ambitious goals, they are opposed to each other and compound the stress of her daily life.

I know many Cathys. Are you one of them? Narrow your focus, or you're going to get nowhere. Do you want to be lean? Or strong? Or do endurance races? Because most people can't do all of them *and* hope to be healthy while accomplishing all that, especially while working full-time.

Does the risk outweigh the benefit?

Not every exercise is appropriate for every person. Just because it looks cool doesn't mean it's right for you. Make sure you have the right strength, flexibility, and control to do an exercise safely. Gymnasts who do work on the rings take years to build up the strength in their ligaments and tendons so their shoulders don't rip apart. Just because you have the strength to do ring workouts doesn't mean you should jump into it with reckless abandon. Sure, you might look cool doing kipping pull-ups or ring dips, but are they worth a nagging shoulder injury for the next two years? Make sure you do the appropriate progression to do the exercise safely.

Will the exercise produce the results you want?

Kay lifts weights often, sometimes for up to two hours, but wonders why she can't lose weight. Once I figured out that her weights were way too light, I was able to shortcut her workouts. She was only lifting one to three-pound dumbbells on every exercise because she didn't want to get bulky. Low-intensity workouts produce low-intensity results. Most of us need to start at low intensity to build a foundation for more intense exercises, but we need to keep working harder to get better results.

Are you overusing muscle groups?

While I love the idea of CrossFit or similar programs, some trainers have little experience putting workouts together and overdo movements in the same plane of motion. For example, it's not uncommon to see workouts that link box jumps, burpees, and squats in the same workout. On their own, they are great exercises, but linked together, they can overload the hip flexors, especially when they make up the majority of your workouts.

A good workout will create balance and symmetry in the body, rotating muscle groups and planes of motion that the exercise is done in.

Is this exercise applicable to life?

Sure, it's great that you can stand on a wobble board and do a kettlebell bicep curl while squatting on one foot, but how does that translate into your job or your life? If it helps you practice the same movement you need to save kittens from trees, then by all means, keep doing it. If you have no idea how to apply the movement to your life, you may not need to do it.

Can you do the exercise in a variety of positions?

Exercises that can be done in multiple positions or planes of motion tend to be more effective than ones that can only be done in a static position. If you started with a seated shoulder press, as you got better, you could progress it to a standing position. Or you could adjust your seat position back so that you do the shoulder press in a different plane of motion. These would all give you slightly different results.

Is this exercise feasible in your workout environment?

You might see a cool new exercise in your favorite fitness magazine and want to try it out. Is it realistic for the environment where you work out? What kind of space or equipment is needed, and how much noise does the exercise create? Some gyms have a policy that prohibits dropping weights. If you're lifting weights so heavy that you need to drop the bar, it may not be an ideal exercise for your gym environment. Either you need to pick a new gym that allows you to drop bars or you'll need to lighten up the workload.

Do you enjoy the exercise?

Chances are that you'll stick with an exercise much longer if you actually like what you're doing. Find exercises that you get some pleasure from so that you do them consistently. I don't always *love* every exercise I do. Sometimes, I do it because I want the benefit or result it produces, but

I know that when I'm doing workouts I like, I'm much more likely to keep doing them.

Dealing with Pain and Injury

The point of exercise is to strengthen your weakest link, but sometimes, that weakest link prevents you from being able to exercise at all.

If there's anyone who knows about injuries, it's definitely me. I'm almost starting to lose track of the number and different types of injuries I've sustained—it's more than two hands' worth. And I'm still pretty young!

Until recently, I didn't understand why I kept getting injured. Until, that is, I learned that I am hypermobile. This makes me kind of like Gumby: extra stretchy and more prone to injury. Since I'm also super competitive and love to push my body to the limits, this hasn't proven to be a good combination. It's resulted in rolled ankles, muscle and tendon tears, and overuse injuries much more than most people. Maybe one day I'll learn!

I've spent hundreds of hours in physiotherapy to rehab injuries, doing icing, stretching, and at times, being laid up, unable to do much. So, because of having so many injuries, I know what it's like to have pain. Sometimes, the pain is there all the time, and it can get frustrating being limited from activities that you really want to do. It took me a while to learn this concept, but I want to share a secret with you: You can *always* do *something*.

Focus on what you can do, not what you can't

I've spent far too much time saying, "I can't exercise because I'm injured," but that's just a giant excuse. So, I'll say it again: Focus on what you can do, not what you can't. If you have a lower body injury, work on your upper body. Hurt your arm? Work on your legs. Have a back injury? Focus on small core-strengthening exercises that you can do while laying on your back. There is always something that you can do to improve your muscle strength, balance, posture, or flexibility. Be creative and start moving!

For most people, injuries happen because of tightness or imbalances. Tight muscles shift your posture or cause you to develop pain so that you use your muscles differently. Joint stress then develops from improper coordination or firing between muscles, causing the injury.

What you might blame as the "cause" of an injury is often a silly little thing like bending over to pick up a pen that causes your back to go out. Or doing the same shoulder press you've been doing for a few months that suddenly wrecks your rotator cuff. In reality, the injury is from the accumulation of years of bad posture and/or tightness. This improper load on your body (especially over years) causes the injury, not necessarily the excess weight you carry or the activity you do. I'm not telling you to stop exercising and get fat! What I do suggest is to correct your mechanics to prevent injury in the first place.

If you have pain during exercise, start with a reduced range of motion on any exercise that uses the muscles or joints near the injury site. Lighten your resistance as much as possible in the initial phases of rehabilitation, so that you aren't stressing the area more than necessary. Gradually increase the range of motion as long as you are able to perform the exercise without pain.

Another way to adjust the exercise while you are injured is to change the plane of motion that the exercise is performed in. For example, a bicep curl is typically done standing up. If that irritates your shoulder injury, you could try it lying on your back with the back of your arms supported. Although it's not an ideal position, it may help provide initial stability to safely progress to the next phase of rehabilitation.

Keep in mind that everything in your body is connected through the network of fascia (pronounced *fash-ah!*) in your body. It's kind of like saran wrap that surrounds all of your muscles, keeping everything in place. Tightness in one area may cause pain in another area. Nerve pain also behaves in the same way. A pinched nerve in your neck may cause pain in the arm. A nerve that's pinched in your back may cause pain down your leg. It is important to diagnose the underlying cause of your injury or pain to prevent it from reoccurring.

How can you prevent injuries? Start with your posture! Stand in front of a mirror with only your undergarments on (or naked, if you really want!) and look at your body alignment. Are your shoulders even? Are your hips even? Even better, get someone to take pictures of you from the front, sides, and behind so that you can really look at them. By being aware of your positioning, you can start to change it. If one shoulder always sits higher than the other, you'll need to pay more attention to bringing it down.

Do you always sit on one hip? Or carry your purse on one side? Perhaps you drive with one arm propped up on the window. These patterns and habits develop imbalanced muscles over time. Stop doing those silly habits! I know—easier said than done, but it's well worth it in the end!

The next best way to prevent injuries is to ensure that you are able to move the way your body was intended to. This is pretty difficult for most of us to do because we are sedentary far too often! If you are not able to move your body through the natural range of motion of each joint, it's likely because your unknown or subconscious bad habits have reduced these ranges of motion over time. Or it's possibly from excess weight. Either way, you can do something about it. Your body isn't meant to sit all day or walk all day or do *any* one specific movement all day. You're also not meant to be in shoes with heels all day or wearing constrictive clothing that makes you walk funny.

Just like when you have an injury, start with a small range of motion for each joint and gradually increase as you are able. Once you are at full range of motion, add resistance at a gradual pace. Rather than jumping aboard the "minimalist footwear" bandwagon, gradually reduce the support or structure from your footwear to allow your foot to relearn how to do its job. If you frequently wear tight skirts that make you walk funny or tight jeans that make it hard to bend over, give your body a break, at least on evenings and weekends, to move normally.

To protect yourself from further injury, progress your exercises more slowly than you think you need to so that these imbalanced muscles have time to adapt. If you do a lot of computer work, your chest, neck, and shoulders are going to be tight and shortened. Your exercise routine should focus on countering this, doing more back exercises like rows, lat pull downs, or chin-ups, along with stretching and opening exercises like a doorway stretch or lying on a foam roller with your arms out to the sides.

Think of your fitness like a pyramid. The bottom is your base of fitness. The broader the base, the taller your fitness pyramid can go. As you rehab from injury, focus on low-intensity exercises for a longer period of time to build a solid base of endurance. This is not the time to focus on the top of your pyramid—your elite level of fitness. Instead, focus on your weakest link and strengthen it so that once your injury is healed, you'll be more balanced getting back to what you love to do.

Chapter Fourteen

A Word on Weight Loss

*S*ince weight loss is such a common topic, I can't really pass on including a section about it in this book. Almost every client I've worked with has had unrealistic expectations for weight loss, thanks to all the marketing of diet pills. Normal weight loss rates are only one to two pounds per week. That's it!

Losing eight to ten pounds per week is not normal, and it's also not healthy. The faster you lose weight, the faster you'll gain it back. Men typically lose weight much more quickly than women, so unfortunately, most women I've worked with end up losing closer to one pound per week. Add menopause into that equation, and it can slow things down even more.

You also need to stop considering using super low-calorie diets or diets with injections—they both completely wreck your metabolism in the long run. These kinds of diets lead to the yo-yo effect of up and down weight that puts unnecessary stress on your heart. To boost your metabolism and burn more calories, keep as much muscle mass on your frame as you can with age, especially for women going into menopause. I suspect this may be a *magic bullet* of sorts to help prevent unwanted weight gain through menopause.

Another common misconception is that if you can burn off calories, you can get away with eating junk food later on. It's amazing how few calories you actually burn compared to what you eat. Abbey started a walking program and wasn't sure why she hadn't lost any weight. Her walk seemed to be an appropriate length and intensity, but she wasn't seeing the results. Once I figured out she was stopping for a hot chocolate in the middle of her walk, it made more sense. She was drinking more calories in the hot chocolate than she was burning on the walk.

Don't use your exercise to excuse calorie intake. Exercise is to help reduce the natural physiological changes your body is going to throw at you, to have fun, and to feel strong and healthy. Most people also don't need to take in extra calories or electrolyte drinks to compensate for their workout unless it's getting to be longer than an hour of intense sweating. These *recovery* products are highly promoted but are not needed for your average workout. They contain far too much sugar and more calories than the amount of energy you just burned off. If you do sweat a lot, consider using unsweetened electrolyte replacements or add a pinch of salt to your water.

For weight loss, I also tell my clients to not focus solely on the scale. Although the scale is great to tell you what your absolute weight is, it doesn't give the full picture. Debbie was frustrated that she wasn't losing weight despite a big effort to lift weights and eat a well-balanced diet. I started to ask other questions and discovered that Debbie had reduced the size of her pants by two and had much more energy than when she'd started. She just hadn't seen the results on the scale because she was gaining muscle mass and losing fat mass.

Since muscle is denser than fat, the same weight takes up less space. This explains why some people can look leaner (skinnier) and stay the same weight, like Debbie. Focus on other results beyond the scale, such as your waist circumference, body composition, mood, or energy. Other people see improvements in their sleep, a reduction in stomach bloating, less frequent colds, and improved skin appearance.

Another way to notice an improvement in your fitness is to track your recovery heart rate. As you get into better shape, your heart rate will

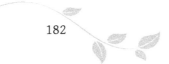

return to its resting state faster, and you'll be able to do a more intense workout at a lower heart rate. These are both signs of improved cardio-vascular fitness—signs you are getting into better shape!

Everyday Fitness

You're convinced you want to start working out, but like most people, you don't think you have the time. The current exercise recommendations suggest doing 150 minutes per week of exercise. I find that for most people, this is far too much to start with. It seems unachievable, so why bother even trying, right? I'd rather start you off slow, build success, and then go from there.

Start out with a quick workout that you can do in ten minutes every day to work toward reclaiming your fitness and getting you back on track. Although a ten-minute workout each day won't turn you into an Olympic athlete, it will help you develop health habits and allow you to start doing other exercises as you get stronger.

Imagine if you only did ten minutes each day. How many minutes would that add up to over time? That's 3,650 minutes over a year and 608 hours over a decade. I think that you could completely transform your body by doing 608 hours of exercise. Does that motivate you yet? It should!

Here's the Plan

You can literally roll out of bed and immediately do the following plan to get your body going at the start of the day. I prefer doing it first thing, as that's when I have the most willpower and am least likely to make excuses for why I can't work out. Start with:

1. **Intense Cardio: 5 minutes**

   Begin your routine dressed in layers, so that your body warms up quickly. Get your heart rate up, so that you are out of breath and start to get a little sweaty. What's "intense"? That depends on your level of fitness. This can be as simple as walking up and down your stairs a few times, or it might mean jumping on your stationary bike or treadmill and starting at a brisk pace. Wherever your current fitness is, is just right! Do what's intense or challenging for you at this moment. It may even vary from day to day!

2. **Rehabilitation Exercise: 1 minute**

   This is your chance to strengthen your weakest link. Work on your problem areas—those spots that are chronically tight or sore. Use a combination of stretching, rolling on a foam roller, cupping, or any other active technique that helps you to fix those weak spots. Try doing exercises for those smaller muscle groups that you tend to ignore. Not sure what to do? Google "(body part) + rehab exercise" and then click on videos. You'll have no shortage of ideas to work on! You can do this to find ideas on all the other exercises, too.

3. **Spinal Mobility: 1 minute**

   Your spine is meant to rotate, bend, flex, and extend. Most of us end up with rigid, locked up spines because we don't maintain the natural movements it was designed to do. It is important to progress slowly in this area, as suddenly increasing your range of motion may lead to injury. Work on increasing your spinal range of motion over time. Consider doing posture exercises or movements that help the spine roll down/back up to gradually increase mobility.

4. **Balance Exercises: 1 minute**

   I've already labeled this one as a "use it or lose it" activity. Do things that help to increase your balance on progressively unstable surfaces. For added value, you could even combine this with other exercises you are already proficient at doing.

5. **Strength Exercises: 1 minute**

   Each day, pick one key exercise that you do for one minute to build muscle mass on your body. It can be a bodyweight exercise (e.g., pushups or pull-ups) or weight lifting (e.g., squat, bench press), lifting a heavier weight. Rotate between upper and lower body exercises to help with muscle recovery and to strengthen your entire body.

6. **Core Exercises: 1 minute**

   You've probably heard that core exercises are good, but you may not fully know what "core" means. Your primary core includes your abs, back, diaphragm, and pelvic floor muscles. I think it's also important to include your bum muscles (glutes), hip flexors, and hip stabilizers in this category. Bridging or planking exercises are highly undervalued and can do wonders for helping people with back pain. Search for new and interesting ways to work your core muscles—just be sure to start simple before you progress to complex exercises.

Once you've finished this ten-minute workout, you can get on with your day and feel good about what you've accomplished. It will help you to develop healthy habits while you get stronger and balance out your body. Feel free to do this two or three times per day for more added value, or do more than one minute in each section as you get stronger. Most of all, do exercises that are fun and keep you wanting to do more!

Maintaining an Active Lifestyle

Rather than exercising to lose weight or create a quick fix, choose to be active as a lifestyle change. You'll be able to stick with it much longer, and you will see better results in the long run. Incorporate activity and healthy eating into your daily life by making it enjoyable and stress-free. Here are some handy questions to ask yourself when you are considering changing your habits around exercise.

Goal Setting

Why do you want to exercise? What is your deep, personal motivation?

These reasons need to be important only to you—not your spouse, parents, or friends. No one can make you do this; you have to be the one to put in the hard work, so find out what tugs on your heartstrings. What reasons hit on your raw emotions? The more authentic these reasons are, the more success you will have in achieving your goals. For example: Lose weight because *you* want to be healthy enough to see your kids grow up, not because your spouse nags you about it.

I want to exercise because: ....

I want to lose weight because: ....

What can you do as a result of exercising? Think of all the things you'll be able to gain by being leaner, stronger, and more flexible. What will you be able to do because of all of those benefits?

Because of exercising, I'll be able to: ....

When I have lost the weight, I will be able to: ....

By losing weight, I will gain: ....

Habits

My current exercise habits include:

The number of days I work out each week are: ....

My dedicated rest days are: ....

My current level of activity is ...., and I have been this active/sedentary for .... days/months/years.

Where to Start

To continue with exercise, you'll want to find something that you either like or can at least tolerate. It helps to look back on the past and see if anything has worked particularly well for you. If you were one of those kids who was traumatized in gym class, there are plenty of other exercises out there that don't involve balls flying at your head and won't cause you to get yelled at by the gym teacher. Just start trying things, and eventually, you'll find something that sticks.

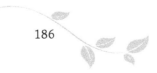

What exercises do I/did I enjoy? ....

What exercises have I always wanted to do? ....

What skills do I need to develop to do this exercise? ....

Break it down into steps to be successful. For example: "I've always wanted to ski, but I weigh 300 pounds and will hurt myself if I go now." To get there: Do exercises to increase endurance, adjust diet to lose weight, do strength training to improve joint stability, take dry-land ski training to target specific muscles, take ski lessons, and progress to skiing. (Timeline? One to two years.)

How much time can you realistically commit to your exercise? It's better to under-commit and be able to do more than to over-commit and constantly disappoint yourself.

I can commit to exercising .... minutes every day. Therefore, I need to work out at .... intensity.

Timing is another thing to consider to help you be more consistent in making your workouts happen. When are you more successful at doing your workouts? (Morning, after work, etc.)

I will schedule my workouts for: ....

Other thoughts to consider:

Do you have access to any exercise equipment?

How supportive is your partner of your new habits?

Do you have any other barriers to changing your habits?

Start by thinking through all the things that might get in the way of working out. Rather than using them as an excuse to not exercise, problem-solve how you can get around them and start moving your body. Have fun!

Pillar 4: Mental Health

"It is during our darkest moments that we must focus to see the light."

—Aristotle Onassis

"About a third of my cases are suffering from no clinically definable neurosis, but from the senselessness and emptiness of their lives. This can be defined as the general neurosis of our times."

—C.G. Jung

"We cannot be more sensitive to pleasure without being more sensitive to pain."

—Alan W. Watts

"Not until we are lost do we begin to understand ourselves."

—Henry David Thoreau

Chapter Fifteen

The Five Ps of Mental Health

Through my work as a nurse and coach, I've noticed that mental health issues such as depression and anxiety seem to be connected to five key components of mental health. By addressing these key components, I've been able to positively impact many lives and get clients feeling better without the use of prescription medications that have many side effects. Those five key areas include People, Pleasure, Pauses, Purpose, and Positive self-talk. I'm going to show you how to create better balance in your life by restoring balance to these areas.

People

The people in our lives contribute to relationships and other interactions that keep us balanced and levelheaded. They provide intimacy and physical touch, which are important psychological needs. If you remember Maslow's hierarchy of needs from Chapter Three: Sleep Essentials, the needs of belonging and love fall in the middle of the pyramid. In the same way that you *need* to sleep, you *need* to have physical connection to others. Babies that are left without physical touch fail to thrive despite their other needs being met. Your needs are no different.

Some people are much more touchy-feely than others. You know the type: someone who just wants to hug you, rub your arm, or sit super close to you—all the time! These people thrive on constant contact and connection. You might think that's completely opposite of how you operate. You need your personal space and don't really like being touched. While there are definitely different personality types, we all need some form of physical connection, just more or less of it depending on our innate preferences.

It's also important to recognize that despite the need for some form of social connection, it's not going to change who you fundamentally are at your core. If you are introverted and get energy from being alone, or from being with just a few key individuals, that isn't likely to change. In the same sense, an extrovert would struggle with being limited in their social connections. You are who you are. What is more important is the quality of those interactions and the personal fulfillment you get from them. Fewer, more intimate connections are likely more beneficial than numerous acquaintances.

Regardless of your personal preference for the type or amount of social connection, there is something magical that happens when we are in the same physical space as others that just doesn't occur in conversations over technology. Being in the same space, your body is able to sense pheromones and other tiny electrochemical messengers that pass in the air, giving you an instant feedback about the person you are near. Sometimes, that comes across as a gut feeling telling you that you don't like that person, and other times, it's an instant positive connection. You aren't able to sense these same chemicals when you are having a digital conversation. This may be part of why humor is often lost over text.

In a world of *instant friends* through various social media platforms and numerous television shows to choose from, people often end up feeling lonely or isolated. They are craving that chemical connection. When someone's pheromones are attractive to you (sexually or not), your body releases a hormone called oxytocin. It plays a role in social bonding. Oxytocin is the feel-good hormone that makes people have some type of intimate connection or even fall in love.

By being in the same physical proximity as someone you feel connected to, your body produces a small amount of oxytocin, strengthening your bond. This release of hormones does not happen when connecting through social media, even if the conversation is the same.

Chatting through technology is an empty social connection not unlike eating empty calories. You can sustain life by eating poor-quality, highly processed foods, but you won't thrive. In the same way, you *can* survive by having interactions through technology alone, but you won't be able to thrive the same way you would if you had a direct physical connection.

If I were to ask you if you are lonely, there's a good chance you'd say no. Most people wouldn't describe themselves as lonely, but upon further probing, many would probably agree that they have some element of loneliness in their lives. As humans, we are social creatures who originally came from tribes and other forms of closely knit communities.

As technology rapidly changes, we are becoming more reliant on using various forms of technology on a daily basis, and our amount of real face time is dwindling. It's no wonder that divorces have become more common and extramarital affairs are going up—we are *craving* connection, even if it means being unethical to get it. Other ways to fill the craving for social connection are through food cravings, self-stimulation, or self-numbing.

Karen was quite introverted and struggled with making friends. She ended up staying home and eating on the couch while she watched TV because she was lonely. By the end of each night, she would overeat on dinner and then polish off a large bag of chips without even realizing it. This habit started happening more often. As a result, Karen gained weight, which lowered her self-esteem. She started feeling bad about herself and didn't want to go out, even when she was invited. So what did Karen do? She stayed home and ate!

Does this sound familiar? The cycle repeats itself just as it does in many of us. I've already given you some strategies for eating healthier. Now, let's look at another way to tackle this.

If you're like Karen, what you really need is a good friend to lean on for support and someone who you enjoy hanging out with. Initially, it can be uncomfortable going out into social situations—this is because these situations are unfamiliar and outside of your comfort zone. You'll want to position yourself for success and have realistic expectations. Don't go out expecting to meet your new best friend instantly. Start with a safe conversation such as ordering a coffee and talking to the cashier about the weather. Become comfortable with being uncomfortable.

As you gain confidence, it will get easier to connect with others, especially if you go to places that are in line with your current lifestyle. Stay off your phone so that you're approachable and can build casual connections. Over time, you'll gain skills to build and maintain relationships.

As your social circle grows, you'll learn who *your people* are. You might already know who they are, the people who you connect with most. They may be family or friends, but you feel at home with them. I've worked with many clients who are in abusive or dysfunctional relationships that just sap their energy. Having people in your life is best when they don't add drama or stress. Ideally, your people support positive relationships and push you to be your best self.

Here are a few thoughts for you to evaluate the relationships in your life:

▷ Who are your closest friends/family members?
▷ Are they there for you without any expectations in return for their friendship?
▷ Do they bring positive energy into your life? Or do they sap your energy?
▷ Are there any relationships you would like to change or end?
▷ Are there any relationships you would like to start or develop?

Pleasure

I'm referring to fun, enjoyment, satisfaction, lust for life—anything that gives you pleasure in your day. In your day-to-day life and on a larger scale, you need to be participating in activities that give you pleasure.

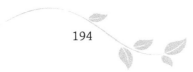

The definition of "pleasurable activities" is going to vary dramatically from person to person. Keep in mind that this section can be closely linked with your connection to people. Participation in pleasurable activities may drive pro-social behavior, encouraging you to surround yourself with people who have similar interests. When you don't have a lot of interests, it can be challenging to be social. The end result is that you often end up isolated without even realizing how you got there.

Savannah is a thirty-six-year-old, introverted engineer and a mother of a fifteen-month-old. She came to me with some complaints about low energy, and she was struggling to lose weight after her first child. After reviewing her lifestyle, I was able to identify that Savannah didn't participate in many pleasurable activities. Like many women, she was busy running around being a full-time employee, a full-time mother, a friend, and a daughter. She really had no time for herself. As a result of her busy lifestyle, Savannah ended up dropping a lot of the fun activities that she used to enjoy when she was younger. Savannah couldn't even tell me what she enjoyed doing because it had been so long since she had done something for herself. She didn't even know where to start.

If you're like Savannah, you are not alone! There are many people who have lost their passions and interests because life got in the way. It's important to go back to things that provide you with fun in your life because they help you to lighten up and give you a broader perspective. Participation in pleasurable activities takes away the need to be serious in every situation all the time.

If you are like Savannah and don't know what you are interested in, you may wonder how you even get started with having things in your life that you can do or might want to do.

A great place to start is by reviewing activities that you used to do or used to enjoy. There's a really good chance that if you've enjoyed activities in the past, you'll enjoy them (or similar versions of them) in the future. So, what activities did you used to enjoy when you were younger? List them here:

....

....

Now that you have a good starting point, how can you start to incorporate these activities back into your schedule? This will start to add pleasurable moments back into your life, giving you greater satisfaction. If you think it's impossible to add those activities back into your day, or you aren't interested in doing them anymore, then it's time to start thinking of new activities that you might like to participate in.

Ready for some brainstorming? Come up with a list of twenty activities that you've never done and think might be interesting to do. The first few ideas might come really easily, and you may struggle with other ideas. Be creative—there are no wrong answers! Come up with anything that you might want to do.

1)	8)	15)
2)	9)	16)
3)	10)	17)
4)	11)	18)
5)	12)	19)
6)	13)	20)
7)	14)	

Now that you've come up with a list of twenty ideas, circle five of them that you are willing to explore further. Find out what's involved in doing them and decide on at least three new activities to try.

Identifying things that might be fun is going to take some practice. The first time you do the activity, you may not love it. In fact, you might even dislike it. So be patient, try lots of new activities, and stick with it to build your repertoire of activities that you enjoy doing.

Pauses

Take a quick pause! What does that really mean? A pause is a break, downtime, interruption, or gap that helps you reset, recover, or rest. We all need some downtime in our lives, and too often we think we are too busy to actually take that break. There are a few different types of pauses that you can take to get some form of rest to help your system reset.

Micro-Pauses

These are the smallest types of breaks. They last between a few seconds to a few minutes. They are tiny chunks of time that serve as miniature resets for the day. These micro-pauses can be as simple as looking up from what you are doing and taking a deep breath before diving into your next task. *Ah!*

Realize that in the greater scheme of things, these micro-pauses don't make a significant difference to your overall mental health, but they do help to keep you focused and prevent you from feeling like a chicken with its head cut off. Micro-pauses help to increase the oxygen in your brain and can be enough of a small break to shift your perspective. Other examples of how to add micro-pauses are walking around your desk, taking a physical pause from what you are doing and then resetting, breathing between tasks, walking to get a drink or go to the bathroom, or doing a quick stretch.

Mini-Pauses

These breaks last between a few minutes to a few hours. Mini-pauses have a slightly greater impact on your rest and rejuvenation. They help to reset hormones and mental clarity, especially when they are performed regularly. Examples of mini-pauses are doing meditation, yoga, walking while practicing mindfulness, stretching, listening to relaxing music, or taking a soothing bath. These mini-breaks can be performed between tasks at work or between a change of activities in your personal life. If you have the type of a job where you need to drive around a lot, your time in the car can be a great time to practice mini-pauses.

Wayne told me that he was highly stressed and struggled with severe road rage. He was always anxious in the car and frequently caught himself yelling or honking at other drivers. He was so wound up that by the time he got to his next meeting, he'd have a hard time relating to his clients. Wayne didn't see the prime opportunity to practice relaxation techniques every time he stepped into his car. It takes intention to shift your perception, but over time, you'll be able to turn a stressful situation into a relaxing one.

Rather than focusing on how stressed, busy, or rushed you are, take these mini-pauses as a prime opportunity to fit in relaxation or stress management techniques. We all have the same twenty-four hours in the day—you can't make that any longer. So rather than me recommending that you add more stuff into your day (because that never goes over well), make better choices about how you spend your time. Take a deep breath to slow down, re-focus, and re-center yourself so that you have energy, clarity, and focus for other activities in your life.

Macro-Pauses

Think big! These big breaks last from days to weeks and are often taken in the form of holidays or vacations. Many people do not use their allotted vacation time. In 2015, 55 percent of American workers did not take their full vacation time. This resulted in $61.4 billion dollars being lost in unused time. The average American taking just one extra vacation day per year would result in $73 billion dollars in economic benefit.

Society as a whole is taking fewer breaks than ever before, and we are paying the price for it with our health. If you are in a job with vacation time (which should be every job), take your vacation! Unless you are building up vacation days to take an epic holiday adventure next year, use your vacation, overtime, and paid time off every year. Only about one percent of this time carries over, so you'll end up losing it otherwise.

By not taking your vacation, you may be increasing your likelihood of experiencing stress, anxiety, or illness. The reduction in the use of vacation time is also costing companies in productivity. You'll be able to get more work done with less effort when you take your given vacation time.

The key takeaway for any type of pause or break is that it needs to be relaxing to you. It doesn't matter what I find relaxing, it matters what you find relaxing. So if you know that meditation *should* be beneficial but you can't wrap your head around doing it, then don't. Or try different types of meditation before you write it off forever. With the availability of so

many free apps, search various topics on relaxation or meditation to find one that works for you.

There are many different types of relaxation techniques, and some just aren't going to work for you. Maybe you like soft, fluffy imagery to help you relax, or perhaps you'd prefer listening to a structured, formal relaxation technique. There are also watches, phones, and computer programs that cue you to practice relaxation at various intervals to help you slow down and rebalance your day. Since there is such a wide variety of tools available, find something that works for you and do it regularly.

As with other strategies presented in this book, it's about *slowing down to go faster.* This is a concept that seemed absolutely absurd to me when I first heard about it. I actually thought the person made a mistake in what they were telling me. Slow down to speed up? When you take breaks, you are more refreshed and more energized. And guess what goes up? Your productivity! If you are more productive, you'll be able to get more work done with less time and less effort. That sounds like a great win, doesn't it? The more you take breaks, the more you'll be able to increase your productivity.

Purpose

It's really important to give your day and your life purpose. Now, inherently, I believe that there's a lot of pressure in the concept of *life purpose.* People get overwhelmed, saying, "I have no idea why I'm on the Earth or what my life purpose is," and that's not what I'm talking about. While it might be great to have a really lofty life goal or a life purpose, it's not essential in this area. What you do need to have is a reason for moving forward with your day or your life that gives you a perception of value. Here are a few examples of clients I've worked with who have different ideas regarding clarity of purpose.

> *Karen wants to go back to school to finish her high school diploma so that she can become a professional stylist. After getting*

pregnant at the age of sixteen, she had to drop out of school. Being a single mom, Karen struggles to pay the bills and isn't sure how she can take care of her son and go back to school at the same time.

—Karen has a clear purpose driving her, but she's currently not sure how to fulfill that dream.

Harper wanted nothing more than to be a mom. Despite having two university degrees and a professional career, she wasn't fulfilled. After having children, Harper continues to work but cherishes her family time. She loves having playtime with her kids and partici- pating in local community events with her family.

—Harper is very clear on her life purpose and is actively engaged in activities that feed her life purpose.

Maria has been retired for fifteen years and became quite isolated. She lives in a retirement building where she doesn't need to cook her own meals or go grocery shopping. Maria doesn't really like the company of the other residents, commenting that they are too old and she has nothing in common with them. As a result, Maria spends most of her days sitting in her own apartment watching game shows on television.

—Maria has little purpose or drive and as a result has become quite withdrawn.

Your individual purpose is what gives you drive or get-up-and-go so that you have a reason to get up in the morning. Purpose can be relat- ed to career goals, education, moving up the corporate ladder, or even starting your own business. Personal purposes may be related to raising children with good values or morals. Maybe you want to be the best mom ever and help support your children to be successful adults. Or maybe your purpose is to support others. You've got a grand vision to change the world with a new product that doesn't even exist, and all your efforts and energy go to pursuing that dream. Or perhaps your current goal is to de-clutter your house so that you can downsize and have a more carefree

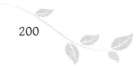

lifestyle. Regardless of how big or small your purpose is, it's important to have something that gets you up in the morning and gives you the incentive to participate in life.

Positive Self-talk

How many times in a day do you tell other people how inadequate they are? How much they've disappointed you? Or how big of a failure they are? Chances are, you don't. You likely keep most of those thoughts to yourself so that you don't offend the other person. It would be inappropriate and mean and would likely hurt their feelings for no reason. Yet I guarantee that you do this to yourself many times a day without even being aware that you are doing it.

Positive self-talk greatly influences your mental health, simply via your own perspective. I'm not a big believer in the *think positive and you can achieve anything* mentality; however, your outlook will greatly impact the outcome and the types of people and energies you attract into your world. Positive self-talk helps to build confidence, self-esteem, and resiliency.

For optimistic people, positive self-talk is much more natural and comes easier to them than it does to others. If you are naturally pessimistic, you're more likely to have negative or self-defeating thoughts about yourself. These thoughts penetrate your world and, on a deeper level, tell you that you aren't good enough, deserving, or worthy.

Keep a journal for one day and write down every single thought that you have about yourself that is negative. I don't care how silly it is or if it's only a little bit negative—or even if it's said as a joke—write it down!

Stop here until you do this activity.

Now that you have completed a journal, count how many times you had negative thoughts about yourself in one day. If you only have a few, then you are doing really well. The higher your number, the more work you have to do to change your internal dialogue.

How do you change these thoughts? The first step is to be aware of your thoughts. If you aren't aware of your thoughts, you can't change them. The second thing I want you to do when you recognize that you are having a negative thought is to rephrase it into a positive thought. Sometimes, this feels impossible.

Here's an example. If you look in the mirror and tell yourself that you are fat and ugly and can't come up with a reason that your negative thoughts aren't true, come up with a different positive statement. You could change your focus and tell yourself that you have amazing eyelashes.

Initially, that change in thoughts is going to seem really silly and really fake, especially if you are used to beating yourself up. But what happens is that you are subtly telling your brain, giving yourself messages, that you are good, worthy, and valued, because you are.

By practicing those comments to yourself on a regular basis, you'll be able to do them more frequently and with less effort. This, in turn, will have a positive impact on your self-esteem, self-image, and confidence. These positive thoughts help you to love yourself for who you truly are, rather than focusing on your insecurities and things that you physically can't change.

Keep plugging away at positive self-talk. It will become a regular habit before you even realize it!

Chapter Sixteen

Ready to Change?

I was working with a patient, Bernice, who came to see me with the goal of losing weight. Bernice was carrying at least an extra fifty pounds on her frame and has struggled with her weight her entire life. In addition to trying several different diets over the years and having yo-yo weight loss and gain cycles, Bernice was also dealing with two anaphylactic allergies to foods (kiwi and shellfish). She also had several other less severe food reactions including fruits, vegetables, meats, and dairy. She was tired of being on a roller coaster and wanted to lose the weight for good. Bernice stated that she had been eating healthy and was exercising regularly, and wasn't sure what else to do.

Bernice started out sounding like she was very motivated and said that she would be willing to do just about anything to change her life and lose the weight for good. I collected a history and uncovered that Bernice's healthy habits weren't as consistent as she had implied. Her "daily" exercise of walking for thirty minutes was really only happening on occasion. Her incredibly healthy diet turned out to be eating out or warming something up from the pre-made food section of the grocery store.

Once we started discussing the details of dietary changes to help decrease the inflammation in her body, plus exercise modifications to help build muscle mass, her whole demeanor changed. Bernice started making excuses—without even realizing it. She told me how much she hated cooking. She loathed it. I listened patiently while Bernice went on to tell me that no one was able to help her enjoy the process of cooking. She had taken cooking classes, attended lectures, watched cooking shows, and tried many more attempts at becoming a master chef. She simply despised being in the kitchen.

After this venting session, Bernice said she would be willing to cook but only if the preparation, cooking, and clean-up could be completed in less than ten minutes. Bernice also said that she was willing to exercise but started focusing on all the things that she couldn't do because of injury or preference, ultimately only leaving a few options for low-level cardiovascular activities.

Bernice's response is more common than you might realize. In fact, this happens all the time. Personal trainers, dieticians, doctors, nurses, and other health professionals will get clients who claim they will do "anything" to see results or make changes, only to see the client set up roadblocks before they even get started. In the example of Bernice, I politely gave her the choice: She could put in a greater effort with her nutrition and continue to exercise on rare occasions, she could exercise regularly and keep eating the same way, or she could find some middle ground by making some changes to both diet and exercise, which would help her lose some weight.

However, what Bernice really wanted was some magic fix to lose weight without really having to put in the effort. As much as I would love to wave my magic wand and remove some of her excess pounds, it simply does not work that way. In order to see change, *you* must change. If you keep doing what you always do, you will keep getting what you always get.

Stages of Change

This theory was developed by two gentlemen, Prochaska and DiClemente, and states that there are different stages of readiness to implement

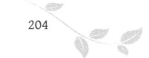

change. It helps to identify how likely you are to engage in a behavior change. Think about where are you right now. How ready are you to make lifestyle changes? Read on to learn more!

Pre-contemplation

This stage is where you are **not** ready. You're not even interested in changing a little and won't consider other options. This is where people often come to me and say, "You need to help my (partner, brother, cousin, friend, etc.) make changes." The frank and honest answer to that is, I can't. I can't make anyone do something that they don't want to do. End of story. They have to *want* to do it themselves before anything can happen.

If you have people you want to help, be especially respectful of their needs in this phase. Trying to guilt them into change isn't going to help them; it's going to create more resistance. So stop nagging them about the change you want to see and start focusing on other ways to build a healthy, supportive relationship with this person so that when they are ready to change, you'll be there to support them.

These people need accurate information on the risks for their disease or condition that they can read on their own time and come to their own conclusions about the information. They need to understand the *why* part of "why should I change?" To help create better buy-in, ensure that this information comes from reliable and trusted sources, not from false media claims, supplement companies, or fly-by-night "health" businesses.

Contemplation

In the contemplation phase, you are starting to think about changes. You likely see the possible benefits of change. You aren't ready to implement real change yet, but you are starting to think about plans for making positive changes.

If you know someone in this phase, it's important to acknowledge the small, healthy choices you occasionally see them making. If you are here yourself, focus on positive self-talk, thinking about the benefits of the change related to your personal situation.

1. What are your personal priorities and goals? By making a change, what will you be able to do that you can't do right now? Or how can you do the same thing with fewer challenges? What are the advantages of changing?
2. Think about your current habits—what risk factors do they create? Do you have a family history of this condition? What are the disadvantages of staying the same?
3. Does your current habit negatively affect others? Is that a problem? What will happen to your relationships if you don't change this risk factor?

I'll cover more on how to weigh the pros and cons of change in the next section. This type of evaluation has a lot of benefits if done in this stage of readiness or during any stage that follows.

Preparation

This is where things start to happen. You've now decided that you want to make some lifestyle changes and are preparing to take action. You have the intention to change in the near future. At this point, you are focusing on your commitment to the lifestyle changes and are spending lots of time finding appropriate resources to help you make changes. You've set goals and are starting to take small steps towards action. Or perhaps your changes are bigger, but you aren't quite consistent yet.

If you haven't done so already, start to develop an action plan. Break down your plan into short, medium, and long-term goals to help keep you on track. Accept that you *are* going to make mistakes. You *are* going to fail. That's what's supposed to happen in this phase. The key is to accept your failure with gentleness and learn from the mistakes you make.

In this phase, it's helpful to start replacing your old, unhealthy behaviors with new, healthy ones. Identify what your triggers are for those old habits and do what you can to remove them. If you always smoke when you have a cup of coffee, you might need to give up both while you are trying to quit smoking.

When you are successful at implementing changes, reward yourself through non-food-based rewards. Perhaps you set money aside to take a

vacation with the money you've saved from not smoking. Or maybe you get to buy yourself a new piece of clothing for every five pounds you lose.

This phase can have its ups and downs, especially since you won't get it right every time. Count on your people or support systems to keep you focused on your goals. Keep putting one foot in front of the other, and big changes will start to happen!

Action

Congratulations! You're now in the doing stage of behavior change. You've been consistent at doing your new behavior change for about six months now and are starting to get the hang of this new way of life. You might occasionally step back to your old habits but are quick to realize it and make a course correction to get you back on track.

This phase also responds well to rewards. How have you planned to reward yourself for sticking with the change? Maybe your reward is how good you feel—the boundless energy that comes with losing that first twenty pounds. Or maybe it's getting to walk your first 5K race. Regardless of what you do, check your progress along the way so that you can see how far you've come.

Maintenance

Once you hit the maintenance stage, you've been successful at implementing a behavior change. You are in the regular habit of doing things the new way, and these new habits have become automatic. You're also able to anticipate when you might have setbacks and can plan for them. This stage is a great time to evaluate what you are doing and how you might be able to make changes to make things run more smoothly. Ask yourself, "What's working and not working in this phase? What can I do to change that?" You may need to identify additional supports or recognize that you need to look at ways to overcome other obstacles that get in your way.

Continue to reward yourself for doing the new habit. This will help to reinforce the positive changes you've made. At this stage, reinforcement can be stretched further apart. Start to focus on long-term goal-setting, as this will give you more to work towards in the future.

Relapse

I used to cringe when I made a mistake. I hated being wrong and making mistakes because it made me feel like a bad person. I took a coaching course that changed all that. It celebrated making mistakes because that meant you were learning how *not to do something.* That brought you closer to finding a better way to do it. Like Thomas Edison said, "I have not failed. I've just found 10,000 ways that won't work."

We will all make mistakes—that's a given! When we can learn from backsliding instead of beating ourselves up over it, we get to see the value in the mistake. So congratulations for failing! Rather than giving up completely, just start where you left off and keep plugging away. Put on your big girl panties and try again! Instead of giving up on your new way of eating because you had a bad night, start fresh the next day. Missed a week of working out? Get back at it the next week, even if it's just ten minutes a day. Relapse is about identifying what you can do about it. Because it's ultimately up to you to get back into your healthy routine.

You'll also want to consider that these phases don't always go in logical or sequential order. They can move around and sometimes skip a phase, moving forward or backward from your current position. Be patient with yourself and just keep plugging away with where you are, with the goal of moving forward when you are able.

The Healthy Decisions Quadrant

Anytime you need to make a decision about changing your habits, there are lots of factors to consider. Sometimes, it can be a simple decision, but when it's not, it can be tough to know where to start. The healthy decisions quadrant helps you evaluate all the good things about staying the same, the bad things about staying the same, the good things about changing, and the bad things about changing.

There are always examples you can come up with for each quadrant, but often, one section will carry more weight than another section. This doesn't necessarily mean that the quadrant with the most answers will win. It's often the quadrant that pulls the most on your heart-strings that wins.

Which variable means the most to you? The variable or variables that really get you choked up, make you mad, or make you want to cry are the ones that have more staying power. That's the quadrant where you're more likely to be successful. Sometimes, that means that you are ready to change, while other times, it means that you've got some work to do before you are ready to start making changes.

How to use the healthy decisions quadrant

4. Identify what your target goal is. Be specific about your goal and write it out on the first line. At this point, you don't need to know how you are going to accomplish your goal, only that you want to do it.

   For example, you may want to quit smoking, lose weight, or start exercising. You would write: "I will lose twenty pounds over the next year."

5. Next, fill out each quadrant to identify the good and bad things about keeping your current behavior, as well as the good and bad things about changing it.

6. The advantages of changing and the disadvantages of staying the same should be more powerful than the other factors. This is so that you'll be ready to make changes. If they are, then you are ready to start working towards your goal.

Example of someone who is ready to change:

Target Goal: I will lose twenty pounds within one year

Advantages of staying the same	Disadvantages of staying the same
▶ It's easy	▶ I am not happy with how I look
▶ I know how to do it	▶ I get out of breath going up stairs
	▶ I can't keep up with my grandchildren
	▶ I may not qualify for travel health insurance next year

Advantages of changing	Disadvantages of changing
I will have more energy	I can't think of a reason not to
I will be more confident in myself	change, I'm just not sure how to do it
I can fit into more of my clothes	
I will have better control of my blood	
sugar, and cholesterol, lowering my	
risk of disease	

Why is this person ready? Their reasons under "disadvantages of staying the same" and "advantages of changing" hold much more value and meaning than the other two categories.

Example of someone who is not ready to change

Target Goal: I will lose twenty pounds within one year

Advantages of staying the same	Disadvantages of staying the same
It's easy	I won't lose the weight
I know how to do it	
I don't have to learn anything new	
My partner does most of the cooking,	
so I don't have to trouble them	
Advantages of changing	**Disadvantages of changing**
I will have more energy	I'm lazy
	I have to cut back on certain foods
	It's too hard
	My family isn't supportive
	I don't have time to exercise/cook

Why aren't they ready? Their reasons under "advantages of staying the same" and "disadvantages of changing" hold much more value and meaning than the other two categories.

Now, it's your turn to try it out.

Target Goal: ....

Advantages of staying the same	Disadvantages of staying the same
Advantages of changing	**Disadvantages of changing**

Ready, Willing, and Able

Motivational interviewing (MI) is a technique for engaging internal reasons to make behavior change and ties closely to the stages of change model we just reviewed. The MI technique talks about the concepts of conviction (the tangible belief that you can change) and confidence (your personal feelings of readiness to change).

I find that clients get confused about these terms, as they can overlap a bit. To simplify this concept, I've borrowed a term we use in the hospital setting to determine if a patient is ready to go home. It's the idea of being *ready, willing, and able*. In order to fully embrace the preparation and action stage of behavior change, you have to be ready, willing, and able to do it. So what does that mean?

Ready

This is where you personally feel ready to do it. It ties to the concept of *"confidence,"* where it's up to you to determine if you feel confident in doing the task. It's the belief in your own abilities. Being ready is more feeling-based and harder to quantify.

Questions to ask yourself:

▷ How ready are you to make a change?
Rate yourself on a scale of 0–10. If you give yourself a zero, that means you have absolutely no confidence in your ability to do the task. A ten would mean that you feel fully prepared and ready to take on the change.

▷ How would you benefit if you decided to change?
Connecting a benefit to the change you're considering will help to increase the confidence in your ability to do it. It will also give you more reasons to stick to your new habit.

▷ What will prevent you from changing?
Thinking about the barriers that *will* happen along the way will help to create a plan to stay on track. Knowing what to do when things go awry will also help to boost your confidence.

Willing

This means that you actually *want* to change. Not because someone else suggested it, but because you genuinely *want to*, for yourself. When you are willing, you actively participate in making the change rather than becoming resentful.

Questions to ask yourself:

▷ Are you willing to make a change?
Rate yourself on a scale of 0–10. A zero means you have absolutely no interest in changing. A ten would mean that you are ready to start changing today. Somewhere in the middle might mean you are ready to make some changes but have stipulations or limitations on *how* you're willing to change.

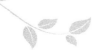

Able

When you are able, you've got all the tools needed to make the change, or you at least know where to find them. This carries over from the term *"conviction,"* the firmly held belief that you can actually do this. It can be measured or observed—you are successful at implementing changes.

Questions to ask yourself:

▷ How confident do you feel about being able to change?
Rate yourself on a scale of 0–10. A zero means you do not think you'll be able to implement the change. A ten would mean that you feel fully convinced that you can be successful at making the change. A rating in the middle means you think you could take steps towards the change, but it may not be perfect yet.

Chapter Seventeen

Motivation

*I*f I had a nickel for every time I've heard a client say, "I need you to motivate me," I'd be a billionaire by now. Motivation is your reasoning behind doing or not doing a certain behavior. It's the desire you have to make a change.

If you need someone to motivate you to do something, it means that you aren't ready to change. You might still be in the contemplation or preparation phase but not quite ready to jump into action.

In sports psychology, I learned about several models that explain why we partake in certain health behaviors. Rather than go through these models in depth (snore!) I thought I'd pull the best information out of them and help you make use of the information they suggest.

Relapse Prevention Model

This model by Brownell, Marlatt, Lichtenstein, and Wilson suggests that approximately 50 percent of people drop out in first three to six months. Sounds a lot like New Year's resolutions, doesn't it? Who really ends up following through on them? Half of you aren't doing the things you set out to do! Some of the reasons for relapsing include having negative emotions, physiological factors, limited coping skills/social support, low motivation, and stress.

Outsmart Yourself:

- **Develop a support network to hold you accountable**

    By having social supports or someone to be accountable to, you'll be more likely to stick with your new activity and create a new habit.

The Health Belief Model

Rosenstock came up with this one, stating that people engage in preventative health behaviors based on the perception of the severity of potential illness or perceived susceptibility to illness. This is a pros vs. cons assessment of your risks. You'll be more likely to avoid activities that you see as risks to your health and to participate in changes that you perceive to benefit your health.

Outsmart Yourself:

- **Identify risk factors to your current behavior**

    This will help you to decide if you are doing things that will negatively impact your health, making you more likely to change bad behaviors.

Theory of Reasoned Action

Ajzen and Fishbein quite simply suggest that people generally do activities that they intend to do. That sounds pretty simple, and it can be. If you plan to work out tomorrow morning, there's a pretty good chance that it will happen, simply because you've made the intention.

Outsmart Yourself:

- **Plan activities to help you achieve your goals**

    By physically writing it down or scheduling a new habit into your calendar, you'll be much more likely to do the actual activity.

Theory of Planned Behavior

This last theory by Ajzen and Madden continues to build on the Theory of Reasoned Action. It states that your perception of your ability to perform a behavior will affect your behavior. In some ways, this is similar

to cognitive behavior theory, where your thoughts affect your feelings, which in turn affect your actions.

Outsmart Yourself:
- **Positive self-talk**

  That annoying positive self-talk rears its head again! Be your own biggest cheerleader. If you don't believe in yourself, who will? You're kind of stuck being with yourself for the rest of your life, so stop beating yourself up and start rooting for the home team. That's you!

- **Speak in present tense**

  Rather than saying, "When I lose weight," talk about things like they've already happened: "I have lost weight." This helps to trick your brain into believing you've already accomplished the goal, making success more likely.

- **Fake it till you make it**

  Yup, that's right. Flat out lie to yourself and pretend to be a leaner, more confident person with more energy—whatever it is that you're trying to achieve. I'm not saying to tell your doctor that you weigh 150 pounds when you're actually 350. What I'm suggesting is that you do the activities you'll be able to do when you lose weight, starting now. Act like you would if you had confidence. Start doing the things you'll do in the future when you have more energy. Eventually, you'll actually believe that you can do it, and you'll become successful at sticking to your new habits.

Barriers to Changing

No one is perfect all the time or always does everything they are supposed to do. I get it. Sometimes, life just gets in the way. But there's a difference between life circumstances and just making excuses for not taking action.

You literally could come up with a different reason each day for why you can't change your habits.

First, as we've discussed already, you have to be ready, willing, and able to change. Once that's set, it's time to remove the common barriers that get in the way of changing. Let's look at some of the most common excuses for not implementing changes.

Time

Time is such an amazing equalizer. We all have twenty-four hours in a day—how you choose to spend that is up to you. So stop using time as an excuse for why you can't exercise, eat healthy, or do a few minutes of stress reduction. You just aren't in the habit of doing it right now, which is why it's not part of your schedule.

You've only got a finite amount of willpower, so use that to your advantage. Do your most important tasks first thing in the morning. If you are trying to get into the habit of working out, do it first thing. If you want to eat breakfast, then plan out what you're going to eat the night before.

- Script out the first 30–90 minutes of your day
- What demands do you have each morning?
- What must you do?
- What will make you feel better for the day?

Attitudes

Do You Moderate or Abstain?

In order to set yourself up for success, it's helpful to know more about yourself and your sneaky habits that sabotage your success. Some people are really good at moderation. These people can eat a few chips, put the bag away, and then forget it's even there. Abstainers, on the other hand, have to abstain completely from eating the food. They can't even eat one chip, or the whole bag will be demolished. For these people, out of sight is out of mind, so it's better to keep tempting foods out of the house.

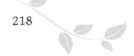

Moderators are better at maintaining balance and can do things occasionally without completely falling off track. Are you better at moderating or abstaining? Plan your lifestyle around this!

Do You Overcommit or Procrastinate?

Some of my clients overcommit. Many of them are triathlon athletes or endurance runners. Whatever I tell them to do, they are going to double or triple it. And just like Tamara (in Chapter Twelve: Components of Exercise and Fitness), this isn't always a good thing.

I heard a great quote: "Good leaders are adders. Great leaders are subtractors." I think that message is really applicable here. Unfortunately, I can't seem to find who first said it—acknowledgement in your honor! The essence of the quote is that not everyone needs to do more. Some people really need to slow down to see better results. If you're going a million miles an hour and aren't seeing results, try slowing down and see what comes of it. You might be surprised by how much more progress you make.

On the flip side, if you tend to procrastinate all the time, you may never hit your goals. If this is your M.O., it's time to step things up a notch and kick it into action. Plan to do the things you *need* to do first, and do the things you *want* to do second.

Excuses

Yup, I've heard every excuse in the book: I don't know how. I have a slow metabolism. I'm big-boned. It's my genetics. I deserve a treat. . . . And on it goes.

When you come up with excuses, what you're really doing is using a cop-out. Quit making excuses and start taking action. Come up with ways to counter those excuses or change your thoughts around them. Sure, you can't change your genetics or bone structure, but that doesn't give you free reign to eat like a pig. You may never be as skinny as you'd ideally want, but you can be healthy with any size or bone structure. Having a slow metabolism doesn't prevent you from being able to exercise; it makes it more important to build muscle mass to boost your metabolism. Find ways to reframe your thoughts.

Money

I can't change what's in your bank account, but I can help you use your money more wisely. Go through your budget with a fine-tooth comb and find out where your discretionary money is going. That's the money that doesn't have to support your basic needs. Sure, you *need* to eat, but you don't *have* to eat at restaurants or buy five-dollar lattes every day. Figure out what your priorities are and direct your funds there.

Sometimes, you'll have to make sacrifices to get what you really want. If you're in a financial group where you truly don't have extra cash to buy high-quality food or buy a gym membership, then you'll need to be more creative. There's plenty of good information on the internet about how to eat healthy on a budget. You can exercise at home for free, and stress reduction can be done anywhere. It's just being creative with how you work to achieve these lifestyle strategies.

Lack of knowledge

This barrier often sounds like, "I don't know how to. . . ." It's not that you don't know how to do something. Anyone can learn how to do something—if they really want to.

Saying that you don't know how to do something is a really lame excuse. It comes down to you being scared, nervous, lacking confidence, or being afraid of failure. To get around this one, you might need to explore your other feelings around why you are hesitant to learn something new.

If you aren't sure where to start learning information about health, reading this book is a great first step. Once you've got a solid foundation of knowledge, you'll be ready to start taking action. What other resources do you need? And where can you get them? Gather up the appropriate resources and supports to get started making healthy behavior changes.

Balance

Okay, I'm sure you've heard about this mysterious thing called balance. But I'm not talking about physical balance in this chapter—I'm talking

about the metaphorical balance you must strike between the pillars of your health.

Let's face it: True balance doesn't exist. At least not in the way that you think it does. Balance is important, but that doesn't mean that everything is equal all the time. I've mentioned that optimal health depends on balance between your seven pillars of health. They don't equate to exactly one-seventh or 14.29 percent of your health. Sometimes, one pillar will be higher or lower, depending on your given circumstances. And that's okay!

This book is here to paint a picture of what things *could* look like in a perfect world. But life isn't perfect. All I ask is that you take the information and strive to be better in each area of health and don't stress about what you can't change. I'm here to encourage you to be a better version of yourself because I believe that we truly can influence a significant part of our health.

I ask my clients to reach for the stars—I've got super high expectations for them, but at the same time, I realize that they aren't perfect. I ask you to do your very best and let the rest go! If everyone made an effort to be only 10 percent healthier, think of the huge positive impact that would make on the health care system. Imagine the burden that would be lifted by your small but noble effort!

So how do you create some semblance of balance between your physical, emotional, spiritual, and mental needs? Between your seven pillars of health? I like to start with whatever area is most out of balance. The one that's creating the most negative impact on your health. If you aren't quite ready to tackle a big topic, perhaps it's better to start with a safe change that can get you on the road to success.

Here are a few questions to ask yourself to help bring better balance in your life:

- How does your current lifestyle affect your balance?
- What areas are in good balance, and which areas need more work?
- What are the advantages of your current situation?
- What are the disadvantages of your current situation?
- What roles do you take on in your life?

- How do these roles enhance/detract from your current health and fitness?
- Is your current situation working for you?
- Is it worth changing?
- Are you ready to change?
- What tools do you need to change?

Balance is a bit of give and take, an ebb and flow of where you chose to give your energy. You cannot be all things to all people. To maintain balance, you'll need to learn to say no. You don't have to please everyone. People are fickle. If you do something to please them, next time they'll want more. Ultimately, you can never work hard enough to make them happy. Do things to make yourself happy and healthy first, then take care of those you love. You'll experience more balance and energy as a result.

Chapter Eighteen

Choose Your Attitude

There's more to choosing your attitude than just thinking, "I feel good," and expecting it to manifest itself. Choosing your attitude is about the mindset that you have going into a new situation.

A Broadway show, *Kinky Boots*, has a wonderful message: "You can change the world if you change your mind." Although their message was related to attitudes around sexuality, I find that it applies to anyone making changes to their lifestyle. You can change your own internal world by changing your mind about how you make lifestyle choices.

Choose to be healthy first and then base your decisions around that. People say, "When I'm healthy, I'll. . . ." But often, health never comes because they aren't making the right choices to be healthy. Why not start with better choices now, so that health can come? By consciously choosing healthy habits, you will become healthy, which will let you do more.

Only you can change your attitude. Only you can take personal accountability for your own health. So regardless of your current situation, it's time that you take charge of why you are in the condition you are in right now. It's no longer your doctor's fault or your parents' fault or your boss, partner, cousin, or dog's fault that you are not well. It's all you. How does that feel to hear that?

This isn't about taking on personal blame for unfortunate circumstances that have happened to you. I'm a big believer in the fact that stuff happens to us that is beyond our control. All of us. And it's just stuff. So it's time to stop blaming others, accept what's going on, and control what you can. There is always something that you can control or change. Your attitude is a great place to start.

I've worked with many clients who feel that they are special, unique snowflakes because they are the only ones dealing with this specific situation. Your situation is likely far more common than you think it is. You'll feel liberated and energized once you can accept that you are the boss of your health and can rule your own world. You can take charge and no longer be ruled by your illness.

If you've conditioned yourself for years that you are helpless, it's going to take a while to change those thoughts. You'll learn to stop being reactive over situations and control your emotional response so that it becomes a habit to make healthy choices.

By controlling my own attitude, I no longer feel deprived when I walk by a bakery with fresh bread. I make sleep a priority because I know how crappy I feel when I don't sleep well. I choose to exercise even on days that I don't want to because I know how amazing my body feels when it's strong. You can learn to do the same thing.

Start by deciding why you want to be healthy. Why do you want to make changes? What are your goals? Then identify the factors in your own life that you can control. You can choose to eat different foods, go to bed earlier, take a few minutes each day to slow down and move your body more, and on and on.

Initially, choosing to do something different can be difficult. Your friends or family might push back. They may try to pressure you to cave in and resume your old habits *just this once*. Stay focused on *why* you are making the decision to be healthy. Then it's no longer a personal decision. You aren't avoiding bread to hurt mom's feelings. You're making choices for your own health reasons. You aren't being deprived. You're in control.

You've had years and years of thinking a certain way. Years to condition a specific belief or thought about how to do things. Simply reading

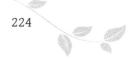

this book isn't going to change that. You have to put in the work. Keep coming back to your *why*, and over time, you'll create a new pattern. What did you learn from your mistakes? From taking the wrong road? Just like that muscle-brain superhighway, you can do the same thing with your thoughts.

It takes time for new thoughts and habits to become automatic. When you are faced with a new decision, or the impulse to resume an old habit is in full force, take a pause. Breathe slowly for ninety seconds. Yup, a full minute and a half. That's enough time to let your brain have its emotional response and allow you to regain your common senses. It will let you make a more logical decision and less of an emotional decision. While you are breathing, talk yourself off the ledge and tell yourself why you are *choosing* to make a different decision. You can say, "I'm choosing to (go for a walk) instead of (eating dessert) because my health goal is to (lose weight). I'm proud of my choice and am in control of my health."

Who's in Charge?

There's a saying that there are three types of people:

Those who do it;
Those who say that they will do it and never get there;
Those who don't want to do it.

Which one are you? Or maybe a better question is, which one do you want to be? If you keep regaining the weight that you've lost, you are doing something wrong. Something isn't working. If you keep *trying* to exercise but never get there, maybe you aren't really ready to do it. So stop saying, "I wish I could be like . . ." and just start doing it. Shift to using your internal locus of control, where you truly believe that you can make permanent lifestyle changes. Because you can. Even if you have to fake it till you make it.

For most people, making lifestyle changes is important but not urgent. Unless you've just experienced a health crisis, it's usually pretty easy to say, "I'll start tomorrow." But stuff gets in the way, and tomorrow never comes. So just like with a bank account, pay yourself first and take care of your health. You can't take care of those around you unless you've got your own stuff under control.

Mental Toughness

Call it mental toughness or hardiness or determination—it's the idea of sticking with change, even when it's uncomfortable. I want you to get comfortable with being uncomfortable. Step out of the victim role and step into a realm of new possibilities.

You may think, "But I've tried everything, and it doesn't work!" So ask yourself, how long were you working on it? How hard did you try? What was your intensity? Did you have 100 percent adherence to your new change? Mental toughness is that stick-to-it-ness that keeps you moving forward even when obstacles get in your way.

To develop more mental toughness, you'll need to put yourself in positions to flex your proverbial mental toughness muscle. You won't wake up one morning and suddenly have the tenacity to conquer the world. You just have to chip away one little bit at a time. Building mental toughness comes with accepting failure. Celebrate it. Yay, failure! What did you learn by failing? Okay—don't repeat that. Try it a different way. Failed again? Great! Now you know two ways not to do it. Keep at it. That's mental toughness!

Having this type of approach will increase your confidence and will increase the belief that you can get through a challenging time. Triathlete Lisa Bentley used to (or perhaps still does) write positive messages on her arm with a permanent marker prior to a race. If she had been struggling with knee pain, she'd write, "My knee feels great." When her knee started aching during a race, she could look at the message on her arm and focus on the positive intention. Lisa didn't become one of the most accomplished Ironman athletes by giving up. She had to push through pain to get there.

While I'm not suggesting that you need to push through injury to reach your goals, you do need to get through some uncomfortable moments to become stronger. Physically, you are capable of way more than you ever imagined. You just need to trick your brain to come along for the ride!

Mindfulness

Mindfulness-based stress reduction is cited in many studies as an effective way to reduce stress and anxiety and improve mood, sleep, and overall quality of life. Some people prefer mindfulness, some people prefer meditation. To me, it just matters that you do *something* to counter all the busyness of your day.

Start with a body scan. This can be done quickly or *really* slowly, depending on how much time you have. Start by taking a few slow, deep breaths. How have you been breathing? Have you been just using the upper part of your lungs? Are you taking short or shallow breaths? Have you been holding your breath? Your breathing pattern can literally shift your stress response.

When you have a short or tightened breathing pattern, your body thinks it's under stress so it turns up those fight-or-flight chemicals. You'll have more adrenaline and cortisol surging through your body, even at rest. Your brain has no choice in this mode but to react using your limbic system. That's the deep inner core of your brain that deals with emotions, motivation, memory, and learning. In this "limbic state," you tend to be very reactive. Your temper is short, you have little focus, and you are more irritable than a hungry bear. Not an ideal state!

By consciously slowing and deepening your breath, you are able to flip back into the rest and digest mode. This helps you to "flip your lid" (ugh!) and get back to using that upper part of your brain (the bulky lobes on top) that help filter your response. These top lobes allow you to be rational in a response instead of being reactive.

Continue to take slow, deep breaths. Where is your energy? Are you tired, energetic, exhausted? Scan your thoughts. What do you feel? What kind of thoughts come up? Are you happy, sad, or thinking of the million things you need to do? Maybe you are calm and peaceful. Is there tension in your body? Where is it? What noises or sounds do you hear? What smells are in the air?

Slowing down even for a few minutes each day to do a full body scan, you'll be able to start noticing when you are tense or not breathing well. A great time to practice this skill is at the start or end of your day. Even better, try both times! You can slip this in for a few minutes between tasks or when you go to the bathroom. It doesn't have to be a huge commitment.

By focusing your attention inwards, you'll be able to gain more clarity on what state of mind you are currently in and will be able to shift your focus. This will help you gain control of your thoughts and feelings, ultimately producing more of the actions you wish to see. Set an intention each day for your health, and check in a few times during the day to see how you are doing. By setting mini-goals, you'll be able to have ways to check back and ensure that you stay on track.

Pillar 5: Digestion

"All Disease begins in the gut."

—HIPPOCRATES

"If there's one thing to know about the human body; it's this: the human body has a ringmaster. This ringmaster controls your digestion, your immunity, your brain, your weight, your health and even your happiness. This ringmaster is the gut."

—NANCY S. MURE

"Laughter aids the digestion. You can eat a huge stew with your schoolmates and digest it with no bother at all, whereas you can get indigestion eating a leaf of lettuce in boring company."

—MAURICE MESSÉGUÉ

"Digestion, of all the bodily functions, is the one which exercises the greatest influence on the mental state of an individual."

—JEAN-ANTHELME BRILLAT-SAVARIN

Chapter Nineteen

Stages of Digestion

The most challenging thing about writing this chapter was knowing that anything I write will become obsolete by the time I published this book. That's because the information on digestion is changing so rapidly that anything we know now will likely change dramatically over the next several years. What I've tried to do, in order to get around this, is to select information that will *hopefully* stay consistent to the essentials and fundamentals of gut health.

Let's start with some basic anatomy and physiology. There are four key steps to digestion: ingestion, digestion, absorption, and elimination. You need to be able to do *all* of these steps well in order to absorb nutrients from food. If you aren't digesting properly, it doesn't matter what food you are putting into your body, you won't get maximal benefit from it. Let's look at a simplified version of each of the four stages.

Ingestion

Ingestion is the process of physically bringing food or liquid into your body by mouth, food traveling down your esophagus, and arriving in your stomach. There isn't a ton of detail that you need here—this is a pretty simple phase compared to the rest. You just need to know that this is how food enters your body. Although you can put substances into your body through other means (injection, absorption, inhalation, etc.) you can't consume food through these means. Now, I admit, some people do appear to inhale their food, but they are really just ingesting it quickly.

Digestion

Your digestive process actually starts in your mouth with your teeth and tongue. You physically masticate (chew) food to break it down. This mixes your food with salivary amylase (saliva) and turns it into a *bolus*—a nice, gooey mixture that is loosely broken down.

Salivary amylase starts the breakdown of carbohydrates. Unlike other nutrients, carbohydrates get broken down and absorbed through the entire length of your intestinal tract.

If you are like most people and eat your food in a hurry, you likely aren't chewing it enough to properly break apart foods, thus skipping the mixing of the key enzyme, saliva. You are skipping an essential step of your digestion! This makes your stomach work harder than it's supposed to.

The bolus then travels down your esophagus into your stomach and gets broken down further into chyme—a pulpy fluid—before it hits your small intestine. Along the way, your pancreas and liver secrete enzymes and digestive juices that help break down food. They focus mostly on proteins and carbohydrates at this stage. Protein is primarily broken down and absorbed through the stomach and upper small intestine—the duodenum and the jejunum. Oh, what funny names our body parts have!

Absorption

A small amount of absorption occurs in the stomach, mostly from fast-digesting, carbohydrate-rich foods. This is why you can see a blood sugar

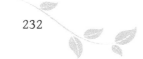

spike so quickly after eating a meal. Most absorption, however, occurs in the small intestine (duodenum, jejunum, ilium), large intestine (ascending/descending/transverse and sigmoid colon) and bowel.

Fat absorption starts much lower down than the other nutrients, happening mostly in the jejunum. The absorption of fat is the most complex of the nutrients (compared to protein and carbohydrates) and much more sensitive to interference from diseases. For anyone who has a problem in this area of their gut, they may experience weight loss. Since fat is the most calorie-dense nutrient, it can be quite noticeable if you aren't able to absorb these calories.

The colon absorbs most of your water, electrolytes, short-chain fatty acids, and about 15 percent of your calorie requirements. These calories come from carbohydrates that have been fermented higher up in the GI tract.

Elimination/Egestion

That's really just a nice way of saying *pooping*. Get used to that word because we are going to talk about poop a lot in this chapter. (You had to know that was coming, right?) This part of your gut includes your large intestine/colon and bowel. This is where you physically eliminate or remove waste from the body.

The Tubes it Moves Through

A typically gastrointestinal (GI) tract is about 480 centimeters long. Changes to this length from internal damage or surgical removal will significantly impact your ability to absorb nutrients and to have optimal digestion.

To compensate for the loss of length, your GI tract can adjust a bit. Your villi (tiny finger-like projections) can actually increase their length, diameter, or function to compensate for the loss of other parts of your GI tract. These villi help to absorb nutrients, so their adaptation is really important in helping to maintain some absorptive functioning. Obviously, they can't make things as good as they were before you had a chunk of your insides taken out, but they can help a bit.

What I find super interesting is that the tube that runs from your mouth all the way through your body to your bum is considered to be an *external* organ. Super weird, since it's inside of us. This part of your body is easily exposed to stuff in the air, chemicals in the foods we eat, germs, bacteria, and a host of other stuff. Kind of makes sense that we have so much bacteria in our gut to help protect us from all of that. But we'll get to that part later.

Advantages of Good Digestion

By being able to do all four stages of digestion well, you'll be more likely to have adequate nutrient production. Your GI tract produces all kinds of nutrients and neurotransmitters such as serotonin. We are learning new information every day about what an important role the gut plays!

Your GI tract is part of building a healthy immune system and is very closely connected to mental health. Your gut produces between 70 and 90 percent of the serotonin in your body, which helps with mood, well-being, and happiness. If you want to have good mental health, improving your digestion is a great place to start.

Dylan is young twenty-six-year-old who has severe bipolar disorder with mixed symptoms of depression and mania. Due to the type of bipolar disorder he has, it has been a challenge to find medication that works consistently for him. As a result, he often needs medication changes and is rarely able to find a balance between his bipolar symptoms and the medication side effects.

When Dylan is manic, he is super impulsive and has difficulty maintaining focus for any length of time. In this state, when he does cook, he often forgets to clean up, leaving his kitchen with unsafe bacteria growing on meat packages or on food that has been left out. When Dylan is depressed and lethargic, he has little energy to prepare foods. He tends to reach for foods that are quick and easy (often very sugary) or the bad kinds of fats. Regardless of his state, Dylan eats mostly processed foods or fast food, with little fresh vegetables, fruit, or lean protein sources.

When you look at Dylan's situation, it's easy to wonder how his gut is connected to this picture. Is his gut not producing the right hormones because it isn't getting the right nutrients, making the bipolar disorder worse? Or is the bipolar disorder preventing the gut from producing the right hormones, which impacts Dylan's food choices?

This is a case of the chicken or the egg. Which came first? Either way, through making better food choices, Dylan was able to better manage his bipolar disorder and reduce the negative impact of his medications.

The Scoop on Your Poop

There is a huge controversy over what a normal bowel movement is. The literature cites anywhere from once every three days to three times a day as *normal* frequency. That's a pretty broad range! More holistic practitioners typically advocate for a poop after every major meal. If you eat three meals per day, you should also poop three times per day. You aren't *technically* constipated until day four of having no poop.

About 77 percent of people are considered to have *normal* bowel movements, 12 percent having hard bowel movements, and 10 percent having loose bowel movements. (I'm not sure where the other 1 percent fall in that study. . . . They have to poop sometime!) This state of *normal* doesn't necessarily mean that it's ideal or optimal, only that it's most common.

While we're on the subject, it's also quite common to pass gas anywhere from six to twenty-three times per day, producing a total of between 500 to1500 milliliters of gas. How they measured that, I have no idea! To put it another way, if you have a few farts a day, you are very normal.

Now, just because I know you love poop so much, I'm going to let you in on a little secret. There is a chart to identify your poo. Who knew? It's called the Bristol Stool Chart, and it explains the different types of poop and classifies them as loose, hard, or normal. So, get comfortable with looking at your poo so that you can use that information to improve your health.

Bristol Stool Chart

Type 1		Separate hard lumps, like nuts (hard to pass)
Type 2		Sausage-shaped but lumpy
Type 3		Like a sausage but with cracks on the surface
Type 4		Like a sausage or snake, smooth and soft
Type 5		Soft blobs with clear-cut edges
Type 6		Fluffy pieces with ragged edges, a mushy stool
Type 7		Watery, no solid pieces. Entirely Liquid

The stools shown between types three and five are typically considered to be normal. They have some form and are semi-solid to solid. They can be sausage or snake-like and are golden brown in color with a texture similar to peanut butter. There should be no identifiable food in these types of stools. The most important part of having a normal bowel movement is that the stool is easy to pass.

Constipation

On the Bristol Stool Chart, constipation falls into types one and two. That's where your poo has separate, hard lumps or nuggets or looks like a lumpy, bulky sausage. The defining feature of constipation is the difficulty to pass the stool—how hard you need to strain to push it out. You can have a *normal* shaped or sized stool that is very difficult to pass.

One of the reasons you might get constipated could be associated with a normal, age-related decline of your GI tract. That is, from a decrease in muscle tone, decreased nerve sensitivity in the colon, or stretching. Other factors may include diet changes, exercise changes, and medication use

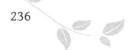

(which tends to increase with age—double whammy!). Some medications that cause constipation are antidepressants, benzodiazepines, iron, and narcotics.

Constipation is often relieved by using medications such as bulk-forming laxatives, non-bulk-forming laxatives, suppositories, or enemas. A more natural way to address constipation is to ensure adequate hydration and fiber intake, along with exercise to stimulate the bowel to move. You can also gently massage your belly in a clockwise pattern (as if the clock were laying on your belly) to help guide your stool in the normal direction of flow. If those methods don't help, try propping your feet up higher so that you can poop in more of a squatting position—this helps mimic a more natural way to go. Don't let constipation go on too long or your stool can get impacted, and you'll have to have it removed through an enema or by manual disimpaction. Neither are fun options.

Diarrhea

Diarrhea is more than just having loose stool. It occurs when you have frequent loose stool and typically ranges between small to moderate volume. This one falls within types six and seven on the Bristol Stool Chart, ranging from mushy or fluffy to completely watery.

Diarrhea affects 5 percent of the population. Although it affects only a small percentage of people, it adds up to $350 million dollars in annual costs from work loss alone. That's a lot of work not getting done because you're stuck sitting on a toilet somewhere. The complications of gas and bloating related to diarrhea can also increase the utilization of health care. Diarrhea can lead to a decrease in quality of life, as it can cause significant stress and anxiety when trying to go out—with the fear of pooping your pants. That definitely isn't something you'd willingly sign up for.

Diarrhea is connected to a host of different causes, including caffeine, chronic infections, food sensitivities, fruit juices, excessive vegetables/fiber, gall bladder removal, increased water consumption, and travel. There are many medications and supplements associated with diarrhea such as antacids, antibiotics, chemotherapy drugs, laxatives (obviously!), magnesium citrate, NSAIDS, and proton pump inhibitors, just to name a few.

Your doctor will want to know how long you've had diarrhea, the type of volume you are producing, what time of day it's present, anything that makes it better or worse, your family history of bowel symptoms, the color of your poop, and if you have a fever present.

To help reduce diarrhea, the best place to start is to identify what the cause is and to remove it if possible. Diarrhea can cause dehydration, so it's important to stay hydrated!

Gas and Bloating

Okay so gas and bloating aren't poop, but they can be signs that things may not be working as well as you want them to. Gas is what comes out as a burp or a fart, while bloating is the abdominal distention or swelling that happens after eating certain foods. Some of the many factors of gas and bloating include:

- **Swallowing air (ingestion)**
- **Foods that ferment in the gut or produce gas**

  The most common foods that cause issues include beans, broccoli, corn, dairy, fruit, potatoes, wheat, artificial sweeteners, and pop.

- **Impaired intestinal transit time**

  This is the time it takes for stuff to travel through your gut.

- **Unable to evacuate gas**

  There may be some type of mechanical (muscle) impairment in pushing out the gas. This could increase gas retention, resulting in bloating and pain. If you are a frequent flyer, this can also happen because of the expansion of gas from atmospheric pressure changes during takeoff and landing.

- **Relaxed abdominal walls/lordosis in the spine**

  Prolonged gas retention can decrease the contraction of your abdominal wall muscles. This relaxation of key core muscles may create an excessive lordotic curve in the spine. (I've often wondered if this is the original cause of men with giant bellies that pull their pelvises forward!)

- **Increased perception of GI function**

    This one may sound silly, but the more attention you give to something, the more you notice it. Think of when you get that nice, new, shiny red car. Suddenly, you start to notice all the other red cars in the same model. They've been out there the whole time, you just didn't notice them before. Symptoms of GI function can be similar. Everyone has gas or bloating from time to time, but the more you focus on it, the more you notice it. There is a delicate balance between ignoring a symptom to give it less power and addressing symptoms because they are problematic. We'll explore this concept in more detail in Pillar 6: Medical Conditions.

So excessive gas and bloating are giving you problems. What can you do to improve your symptoms? There are several ways to try to improve gas and bloating on your own before you rush to the nearest medical clinic.

- **Reduce or eliminate gum, carbonated drinks**

    They may be the primary way you are ingesting gas and are an easy fix.

- **Avoid FODMAPS (fermentable oligosaccharides, disaccharides, monosaccharides, polyols)**

    These come from fermentable foods such as cruciferous vegetables, dairy, fiber fructose, fructans, lactose, legumes, and sorbitol.

- **Exercise**

    Similar to treating constipation, exercise can improve movement of gas and reduce symptoms of bloating.

- **Use probiotics**

  Both *lactobacillus acidophilus* and *Bifidobacterium lactis* are commonly used probiotics that seem to have a positive impact on gut health. There's more information to follow on probiotics!

- **Reduce antibiotics**

  While antibiotics are sometimes necessary, they are overused in our food supply and overprescribed to patients who insist on using them, even when it's not appropriate. Only use antibiotics when absolutely necessary. A common cold or flu does not qualify!

- **Medication/therapies**

  Some classes of drugs called prokinetics can improve the time it takes for food to travel through the GI tract. Others such as Beano or activated charcoal may help to decrease the side effects of certain foods but are suggested to only have minimal benefits.

- **Stress management**

  Just think what happens to the rest of your body when you are stressed. You tense up. Those same tense muscles tighten everything around your gut and potentially even the entire digestive tract itself. (I couldn't find specific research on gut tightening, but it seems plausible to me. You do have muscles along your gut to keep things moving—why wouldn't they get tense too?) To help reduce stress or muscle tension, try mindfulness relaxation techniques, psychological therapy, cognitive behavioral therapy, or hypnotherapy.

Your Microbiome

Your microbiome can also be referred to as intestinal flora, micro flora, or bacteria. It's all of those good bacteria and their byproducts that live inside your intestines.

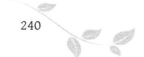

At the time of this writing, it's well known that there are over 500 species of bacteria and 10^{14} (that's 10 with 14 zeros behind it) bacteria in your GI tract. That's a ton of bacteria. You have more bacteria inside of you than all of your other cells combined. I also expect that as we learn more about the gut, these numbers will increase significantly.

Roles of Bacteria

Your bacteria play several known roles in the GI Tract:

- **Immune function**

  Your gut helps with phagocytosis (eating old, useless cells) and preventing nasty things like yeast infections from taking over

- **Mucosal barrier**

  Say what? That's the lining of the walls of your gut that keep the inside separate from the outside. Remember how I said that your insides are actually connected to the outside? Well, you want to prevent the wrong stuff from getting through your intestinal walls to your real insides. The mucosal barrier, when working properly, should keep out tiny food particles or bad bacteria that shouldn't be inside you.

- **Metabolism of drugs**

  Yes, those lovely little bacteria help to break down medications so that they can do what they are intended to do.

- **Production of vitamins, neurotransmitters, and fatty acids**

  Your tiny bacteria are powerhouses for producing thiamine (B1), biotin (B7/Vitamin H), Vitamin K, fatty acids, serotonin, tyrosine, and tryptophan (and probably much more than we can even imagine)

Factors Affecting Your Bacteria

So now you know what your bacteria do. But what about all the factors that affect them? If you have too much or too little gastric acid or enzymes, things can go awry. Compare that to the number of people who are on acid-suppressing drugs for extended periods of time. This messes up the way food is broken down, which has to have an impact on your bacteria.

When your mucosal barrier isn't working properly, microscopic food particles can slip into places they don't belong and cause trouble. When that happens, it's called leaky gut or intestinal permeability, and is due to inflammation or an increase in space between cell walls (which is usually sealed tight).

Enterocytes are the cells in your intestine that absorb stuff that is digested or produced in your gut. Sometimes, they don't work properly or don't turnover at the right rate, adding to poor digestion. Or maybe your gut pushes food along too fast or too slow (peristalsis) or has faulty valves that let food pass along at the wrong time.

That's a lot of stuff that can go wrong. The biggest problem with all of these issues is that you literally have no idea that they are going on. I've never met a person who could say, "Today, my ileocecal valve is operating too quickly," or "my microvilli don't like it when I feed them cheese." We are woefully ill-equipped to make any detailed observation about what's happening on the deeper level of our complex digestive process. Perhaps that's a good thing.

Causes of Dysbacteriosis

Ugh, another hard word to say! Dysbacteriosis is the deficiency or absence of normal bacteria in your gut. You can also have an imbalance, where there's too much of one type of bacteria and not enough of the others. Both of these are bad scenarios. So why would you have these kinds of problems? One of the most common ways is from antibiotic use or antibiotic residues in meat/fish/milk, etc. Antibiotics wipe out all of your gut flora (good and bad), making your gut environment a bacterial desert.

Many diets recommend low or no protein, but protein deficiency can deprive your cells of the nutrients they need to produce mucus in your GI tract. This mucus protects the intestinal lining from the corrosive acids needed to break down your food. Acidity can change from diarrhea

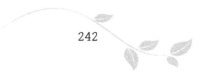

washing out the good bacteria or when you are unable to produce the right number of digestive enzymes (too much or too little).

Other dietary changes, such as adding too much fiber too quickly, can cause food to ferment in the gut, which overwhelms and destroys your bacterial army, leading to gas and bloating. Introduce fiber slowly to allow that bacterial army to build itself up. Some food coloring, such as the purple colors, are believed to kill the good bacteria in your gut. I don't think any food coloring is good for you, but this one appears to be especially problematic.

External sources of dysbacteriosis can come from chemotherapy or radiation. Cancer treatment annihilates anything in its path—good or bad. It's also well known that heavy metals such as arsenic, cadmium, lead, mercury, nickel, and silver can be toxic even in trace amounts. And an obvious cause would be physical changes to the gut from conditions like Crohn's, Colitis, Diverticulitis, and Diverticulosis. In the next chapter, Stuff That Can Go Wrong, we'll discuss the many complications that can affect the digestive system—and how to fight them!

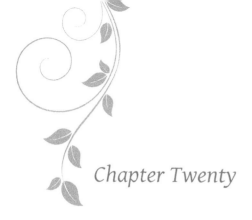

Chapter Twenty

Stuff That Can Go Wrong

Now that you have a better understanding of how your digestive system works, we'll get a bit more in-depth with what might be going wrong inside of you, perhaps without you even knowing it.

What are the consequences of poor digestion?

Poor digestion is when you have frequent constipation, diarrhea, or excessive gas or bloating. Between 10 and 15 percent of the population have symptoms of irritable bowel syndrome, but only 15 percent of those people actually seek medical care. The direct and indirect costs of poor digestion add up to $30 billion dollars annually in Canada alone!

Causes for GI Dysfunction

There can be many causes for GI dysfunction. Some are quite common, while others can be more challenging to identify. I've listed the most common ones here for you. Remember: Common things are *common*—stop thinking that you have some crazy, rare condition. Perhaps you do, but it's more likely something common.

- Malabsorption from lactose intolerance or celiac disease

- Short gut syndrome (Crohn's or colitis)

- Small intestinal bacterial overgrowth (SIBO)

  This can either be from excessive populations of certain bacteria or an imbalance between the different strains.

- Inflammatory bowel disease or syndrome

- Medications (especially antibiotics)

- Dysbacteriosis

Symptoms of Poor Absorption (Malabsorption)

- Anorexia

  This isn't the kind of anorexia where you choose not to eat. It's a complete disinterest in food, ultimately not being hungry.

- Frequent flatulence/gas

- Abdominal distention

- Stomach rumble (the fancy term is borborygmi)

- Nutrient deficiencies

  Despite adequate intake of nutrients, you may not actually be absorbing them.

- Greasy and pale-colored stool

- Excessively large stool

- Foul-smelling stool

  Not that any poop smells like roses, but if you can clear a room with one dump, it may be a sign that you aren't digesting well.

- Asymptomatic

  Some people have no symptoms at all, but just because you don't have symptoms doesn't mean you have good digestion.

How to Fix Malabsorption

It's not all doom and gloom here! Now that I've told you all these horrible things about your absorption, how do you fix it? Here are a few things that you can start with now.

Decrease Your Caffeine

You're really going to start hating me for telling you to give up caffeine. If you have diarrhea, caffeine may be your culprit. Aim for less than one cup of caffeine per day. Give it a try and see what happens.

Increase Your Caffeine

Fooled you! On the flip side, you may tend towards being constipated. If you fall into this category, you might have success in your morning constitutional by drinking a cup of coffee to get the trains running on time. Coffee and poo are friends if you trend towards constipation.

Eliminate Sugary Beverages

Sugar can stimulate the bowel and increase the volume of diarrhea. If you drink lots of juice, electrolyte replacement drinks, or pop, you may get the runs. I don't typically recommend any of these sugary drinks for anyone, so this falls in line with my recommendations in Chapter Five: Nutrition Essentials. About half of the population can't digest fructose, so pouring in fruit juice (instead of eating the real thing) will wreak havoc on your gut.

Supplements

If you have a disease that impairs your digestion, you may need to take between five and ten times the recommended dietary allowance for nutrients just to break even. Breast cancer patients are frequently told to take 5000–7000 IU per day of Vitamin D, well over the normal recommended limits. Those with celiac disease may need additional iron and folic acid. Calcium and magnesium are commonly recommended after bowel resection. The omega-3s have been strongly shown to decrease inflammation, which can reduce diarrhea symptoms. There are many more common supplements with disease conditions, so check with your health care professional to determine if supplementing is right for you.

Remove problematic foods

If certain foods trigger your digestive symptoms, then it's time to pull them out of your diet. These may include gluten, dairy, FODMAPS, fructose, nightshades, or any other list of foods that may cause you issues.

Keep in mind that while these can be quick fixes, they often need to be done consistently to give you consistent improvement in your digestion. If you are lactose intolerant and only have milk once a year, you'll react, clear it out of your system, and move on. But if you're a sensitive celiac, then one tiny speck of a breadcrumb every few weeks can keep your gut inflamed and irritated all year long. You can't just be good 80 percent of the time and expect to fair well. You need 100 percent compliance, no exceptions. These irritants can cause gut issues that you don't even notice until years later.

Many people also have sensitivities to foods like gluten without being diagnosed as celiac. This gets termed as non-celiac gluten sensitivity and is becoming much more common. If you fall into this camp, you are still damaging your gut with occasional exposures to gluten, so it's best to completely eliminate it to prevent unnecessary inflammation.

Other Ways to Improve Digestion

You may not have malabsorption, but perhaps your digestion just seems a bit *off*. There are several things that you can do on your own that can help increase those good bacteria in your gut and to improve overall digestion. Not all of these techniques are right for every person, so make sure that you work with a health care professional to find what techniques are ideal for you.

Chew your food

Seems pretty obvious, eh? (Hey, I'm from Canada! I had to slip in at least one "eh.")

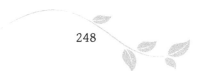

I know your mother yelled at you to chew your food 200 million times, but it's true. Remember how I said digestion starts in your mouth? This is your chance to shine. Chew like you've never chewed before and break down that food well before it goes down. Chew your food slowly. You should even chew liquids that have calories in them. That includes your beloved smoothie, latte, or even soup.

To add even more value to this one, don't talk with food in your mouth—it can introduce unnecessary gas (if that's an issue for you). Wait until you've swallowed to speak your mind. It's also really important to eat when you are relaxed instead of in a rush while you're off to the next thing. Take a slow, deep breath before you take that first bite to remind yourself to slow down. Breathing slowly will help to shift you back into digesting mode.

Process your food

In Pillar 2: Nutrition, we discussed how processed foods are less than ideal. Now, I'm going to try to confuse you. Processing food at home can actually improve digestion without dramatically affecting its nutrition content. The easiest way to "process" a food is to change its shape by cutting, chopping, slicing, or grating it. The next step in processing would be to cook it, which could be done by using an acid (like lemon juice) or by some heating method such as boiling, baking, frying, or barbecuing.

Start out with well-*processed* food by chopping it into little bits and then cooking it well (like a soup or tender stew) or even blending it. You might lose a bit of nutrient content by doing this. Let's imagine that you aren't digesting well, and vegetables pretty much pass right through you. In this scenario, you likely aren't getting much nutritional value. If, by processing your food well, you're able to absorb as little as 10 percent of the nutrients, you still come out ahead.

Slowly reduce your cooking time or the amount you process your food as you become better able to tolerate it. If you notice an increase in symptoms of gas, bloating, diarrhea, or constipation, go back to what you were doing before. If your gut is really broken down, it may take months of this type of technique to get things back on track. Introduce vegetables very slowly, so that you can eventually get a higher intake of plant matter. For some people (with severe Crohn's, colitis, celiac, etc.) this may take months or years. Your patience will pay off in dividends as you're able to absorb more of the nutrients from your food.

Probiotics

When supplementing with probiotics, it's important to continuously rotate the brand and type of bacterial cultures you are getting. This helps to prevent that bacterial overgrowth (as in SIBO) while neglecting other types of bacteria. If you supplement with probiotics, I suggest that you take one bottle and then buy a different brand next time to keep mixing up the type of bacteria you get. I anticipate a huge increase in research in this area and suspect that many new types of probiotics will become available in the next five to ten years.

Yogurt is on the rise as a top source of probiotics. I'm worried that there's much more hype in this than actual benefit. Most yogurt appears to have the good bacteria added before it's pasteurized. That flash of heat is meant to kill any bad bacteria and likely kills all the good stuff they just added. So why does it help you poop? Many probiotic yogurts also contain inulin, a potent laxative that helps you poop. It may not be the probiotic helping you out but the inulin tricking you into thinking that your yogurt is magic. There are likely better probiotic sources of food than the highly processed yogurt in your nearest dairy section. Try out unpasteurized sauerkraut, kimchi, or other fermented vegetables.

Prebiotics

You may have never heard the term *prebiotics*, as information on them is only now on the rise even though they've been around forever. Prebiotics are the indigestible plant fiber sources that ferment in your gut and help to feed your good bacteria. They are foods like garlic, leek, and onions and appear to produce longer-lasting results than probiotics. Don't go crazy and start jamming these foods into every meal. You'll overwhelm that bacterial army and end up bloated. Then you'll swear off vegetables

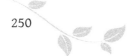

forever and end up hating me. Slowly start adding more prebiotic foods into your diet, just like you're starting to do with other vegetables.

Amino Acids

Back to those building blocks of protein you learned about earlier. An amino acid, L-Glutamine, can stimulate regeneration of your intestinal mucosa. Animal studies show promise in arginine or citrulline to reduce intestinal permeability. Rather than rushing out to buy individual amino acid supplements, perhaps it's just better to eat a wide variety of whole protein sources to help your body do this naturally. Protein is essential for these roles, so if you choose a vegetarian or vegan diet, you may need to sit down with a dietician to ensure that you are getting enough of the right amino acids.

Fiber

The recommended daily intake of fiber for men is 38 grams a day and 25 grams a day for women. Unfortunately, many of us only get 10 grams a day or less, far below the RDA. Start by adding fiber slowly, with the goal to get up to the RDA over a few months. As we've discussed before, dumping a whole bunch of fiber into your system is sort of like pouring a bag of concrete into your system. Make sure that you increase your water intake along with your fiber intake to thin out your potentially concrete stool.

Medications

I've already pointed out medications that can cause constipation and diarrhea. It's well known that medications can change your bowel habits. Make sure that you follow up with your prescribing doctor to remove unnecessary medications. I've seen far too many patients who have been on medications for years when they only needed to be on them for a short time. Save your gut some trouble and get yourself taken off any medications that you no longer need.

Pillar 6: Medical Conditions

"The medical literature tells us that the most effective ways to reduce the risk of heart disease, cancer, stroke, diabetes, Alzheimer's, and many more problems are through healthy diet and exercise. Our bodies have evolved to move, yet we now use the energy in oil instead of muscles to do our work."

—DAVID SUZUKI

"The good physician treats the disease; the great physician treats the patient who has the disease."

—WILLIAM OSLER

"Even if you have a terminal disease, you don't have to sit down and mope. Enjoy life and challenge the illness that you have."

—NELSON MANDELA

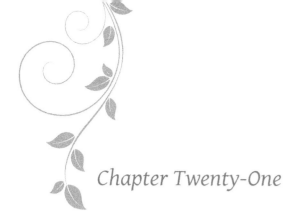

Chapter Twenty-One

Disease Management

M anaging diseases has become the staple of our health care systems. You get sick, you go to the doctor, they treat you, and you
get better, right?

Disease management is so much more than that. Unfortunately, with
our deteriorating health, our health care systems are having a hard time
keeping up with the demand. Regardless of where you live, trends are
showing that health care costs are continuing to skyrocket.

This increase in diseases could be from a number of different factors.
We have increased longevity due to medical advancements, so by living
an extra thirty to fifty years, we are more exposed to opportunities to
become sick or injured. In addition to living longer, we've experienced
a lot of changes over the past several hundred years. We are now exposed to more refined foods, chemicals, pesticides, excessive fats, sugars, salts, increased use of feedlots, and GMOs. To add to that, we have
increased stress, less sleep, artificial light exposure, decreased activity,
and increased antibiotics. All of these factors are likely to play some role,
especially as we pass the effect of these factors along in our genes. It's

likely impossible to narrow it down to just one or two reasons why we are getting fatter and sicker.

As I mentioned in the introduction of this book, the cost of chronic diseases accounts for approximately 46 percent of the global economic burden of disease, and by 2020, that number is anticipated to rise to 57 percent. But instead of just trying to catch these preventable conditions early, we should be using primary prevention to *prevent* them from ever happening.

Lots of programs claim to be aimed at primary prevention, but they are actually doing secondary prevention—where you aim to reduce the *impact* of a disease by catching it in the early stages. Primary care tends to sit in this spot. They do an excellent job of screening to catch diseases early so that they can be treated. This, however, is not primary prevention.

Our health care systems place very little emphasis on primary prevention. How can we change this? First off, only buy products that support healthy living. Engage in activities that help you maintain a healthy weight. Public demand dictates industry. Imagine if tomorrow, everyone stopped buying unhealthy, processed food. Or everyone started going to the gym. The market would have no choice but to respond to the demands we place on the system. The more people demand better quality food, better work-life balance, or cheaper access to exercise facilities, the quicker these changes will occur.

So how do you want to participate in your health? You've got two opposite choices for managing medical conditions, assuming you aren't choosing to ignore the issue altogether. One extreme is to only take medications. The other extreme is to use only diet and lifestyle modifications. Most people land somewhere in the middle.

I've already given you tons of information on the diet and lifestyle end of things, but sometimes, that just isn't enough. Sometimes, genetics take over and throw more at you than you can handle. That's where modern medicine should step in, after you've already done some things to try and improve your chronic illness. This chapter will talk more about the medical management of diseases.

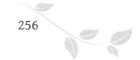

Key Components of Medical Conditions

Diseases are due to a combination of factors including your genetics, socio-economic status, physical environment, and behavior. The more risk factors you engage in, the higher your chance of developing one or more of the major chronic diseases such as cardiovascular disease, cancer, diabetes, chronic respiratory conditions, and mental illness. Well-known risk factors include smoking, an unhealthy diet, being overweight, having a sedentary lifestyle, substance abuse, psychosocial stress, overuse of painkillers, poor sleep hygiene, and unsafe sex. Let's dive a bit deeper into some of those factors.

Family History (Genetics)

Some of your risk factors for disease get passed on to you in your genes. Kind of like the hand-me-down jeans you got from your big sister, they carry the imprint of where they've come from. Genes can dictate the color of your hair, how tall you are, your predisposition to certain diseases, and so much more.

Some families have a strong family history of certain conditions. For example, all the males in your family died before age fifty-five, or all the women developed breast cancer in their early forties. But just because you have the genetic tendency doesn't mean you get to use this as an excuse to not do anything about it.

You've also got epigenetic factors that basically tell your genes to turn on or off. They are the factors that determine if you *express* a gene or not. Kind of like a light switch. The ability to have diabetes is there. Whether you choose to turn that light switch on or off is partly up to you. Some of the epigenetic factors include what type of birth you had (vaginal or C-section), environmental factors during your life, nutrition status, sleep, stress, and other lifestyle factors. While not all epigenetic factors are modifiable, they appear to have a cumulative effect where, at a certain tipping point, certain genes turn on.

You can start by being aware of your family history of disease. Ask family members about conditions that run in your family so that you are aware of what diseases you are more likely to be predisposed to. You should also have a record of all of the clinical diagnoses in your life, past surgeries, and injuries, just in case they're ever needed at a medical appointment.

Medical Management

Despite having a medical condition, it's more about what you actually do about it. Are you following up with your health care professional? Do you get annual health checks to make sure things are on track? Do you know when your next appointment is supposed to be? It's important for you to know and understand your medical condition(s) so that you can manage them properly.

Follow medical advice or seek out alternative options and second opinions, but don't ignore the issue. Screening alone can do wonders for prevention. If nothing else, at least get your annual physical so that you can stay on top of issues as they arise. Conditions like diabetes or high blood pressure don't just go away because you *feel fine*. You can't *will* diabetes away by ignoring it. Many diseases have effects that you can't tangibly *feel* until way down the line. Then it's too late.

To take charge of your medical condition, show up for your appointments on time and be prepared. Get your lab work or diagnostic testing done before appointments so that your doctor has information to follow up on. Have you ever asked questions about what else you could do to manage your care? By showing an interest in your health, your health care practitioner will know that you're serious, and will be more willing to give you extra information.

If you notice that you aren't tolerating pain well, feel frustrated, or have a lack of motivation to manage your condition, ask for more support. It's easy to be overwhelmed by all the things you are *supposed to do* to manage your condition. Especially for patients with conditions like cancer, there can be a lot of information to take in at once and a lot of appointments to attend. This is where your support team comes in. Find out what other services you have access to for support such as social workers or psychologists that can help provide you with better coping skills.

Medication Management

The first thing that I want you to do is to go through your medicine cabinet and pull everything out. All of it! Now I want you to look at the expiration dates and only put back medications that are still current. Seriously—do it now! Taking expired medications can have serious consequences. Some medications may also lose their effectiveness.

Next, compile a list of all the current medications and supplements you take, including the dosage and the reason for taking them. There's usually more than one use for a drug, so it's important to know why you are taking it. Keep a copy of this list in your wallet or in your phone for easy access. In the event of an emergency, it's helpful to have a list of everything you are taking to avoid drug interactions.

If you do take prescription drugs or supplements, make sure that you are taking them as prescribed. It's surprising the number of people who stop taking medications due to the side effects but don't tell their doctors.

Some side effects decrease over time while others may increase. Your pharmacist will be a great resource to help you understand the side effects. Make sure that you consult with a health practitioner before self-medicating (changing it yourself) because some drugs need to be tapered slowly to avoid massive withdrawal symptoms.

Medication costs can be an issue for some people. Find out if a drug plan may be more cost effective for you in the long run. If you don't qualify for a drug plan, ask your health care professional what lifestyle habits could you change to decrease the amount of medication needed.

Can you treat your condition naturally? Making lifestyle changes can be much cheaper than some medications and may be just as effective. Tom was able to get rid of one oral diabetes pill and cut his insulin dose and blood pressure pill in half just by losing thirty pounds. Tom's story is very common. I work with many clients just like him. You can likely do the same if you really want to.

Germ Management

Who knew that you had to manage your germs?

Looking back over the course of medical history, there have been some pretty big changes in this realm. To start, we literally had no idea that germs even existed until relatively recently. Then we became aware of germs and created drugs, hand sanitizers, and antibacterial products to kill them all because we thought they we all bad. Now we're in a phase where we realize that there has to be a balance between good and bad germs. The fancy term for this is antimicrobial stewardship, being more discerning about when and how to use antimicrobials.

As I pointed out in Chapter Nineteen: Stages of Digestion, your gut bacteria are super important. If you are obsessive-compulsive about using hand sanitizers, you or your family may not be exposed to the good germs you need to build healthy immune systems. There's a balance to be had in terms of hand hygiene.

When I work in the hospital, I'm really diligent about washing my hands and using the hand sanitizers. That's because there are some really bad bugs there that should not be spread around. When I'm out in the woods on a backpacking trip, I sometimes forget to wash my hands altogether. I feel like the little bit of dirt on my fingers is probably good for me. Maybe I'm just crazy!

Compounding Factors

There are many other factors that connect to disease management, creating a giant spiderweb of interconnectedness. Socioeconomic status is a huge factor that interrelates with many other factors. Financial status determines the ability to access services and other elements that can positively impact health. Homelessness is directly connected to the access to acute care. And, of course, homelessness is strongly connected to mental health—homelessness contributes to poor health, and poor mental health contributes to homelessness. It's cyclical. You can't just address one issue on its own and expect the whole picture to improve.

When considering these types of complex situations, it's best to look upstream and start with the *cause* of the issue rather than focusing on treating the symptoms. Otherwise, you'll get bogged down in the

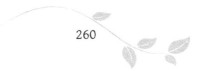

treatment of symptoms alone. Addressing education and mental health issues are usually really great places to start.

Measurement Tools

We are reaching a point where most industrialized countries are having huge issues with weight. Depending on which country you are in, an average of 40 to 60 percent of your population is either overweight or obese. You can see why it's easy to think you aren't overweight when you compare yourself with your peers. Chances are, you look just like your closest friends.

This isn't about fat shaming or chastising people for their weight. It's about what's healthy. Having over 35 or 40 percent of your body as fat is not healthy. I don't care how active you are or what your blood work looks like. Your fat cells are where you store most of the toxins in your body. Higher fat equals higher toxin load. In today's world, with chemicals surrounding us everywhere, that's huge! That doesn't even account for the increased strain on your organs or joints, which takes its toll over time. By being leaner, you'll have better fuel usage, increased performance, and less wear and tear on your joints.

I'm not trying to create eating disorders or make everyone fat-phobic. Being super skinny isn't always better. Skinny doesn't necessarily mean healthy. Some skinny people can still have lots of visceral fat. That's the fat that surrounds your organs and is strongly correlated to disease risk. You also need a little bit of stored fat to insulate your body and protect your organs from damage if you get bumped around—the key word here is "little."

Don't be misled by the excuse that "my fat isn't around my belly, so it's okay." It's about finding some middle ground and an ideal body composition that you are able to consistently maintain over the course of your adult years. So how do you measure these things?

Body Mass Index

As discussed in previous sections, BMI is a metric that contrasts your weight against your height and suggests that risk factors go up or down depending on your ratio. The idea behind BMI is that it's meant to assess your body composition. The WHO supports the claim that as BMI increases, the proportion of medical conditions also increases due to the increase of fat mass. However, BMI is only a tool and has its faults.

In my personal training years, the number of obese clients I worked with far outweighed the normal-weight clients. What their BMI didn't show was that some of these *obese* clients had body fat of less than 10 percent and were extremely muscular—not at all obese. That's the downfall of this tool. It doesn't differentiate between fat mass and muscle mass. It's just looking at your total mass compared to your height. The utility of BMI in athletic populations is not a valid indicator of health.

Most credible sources agree that a healthy BMI is somewhere between 18.5 and 24.9 kg/m². However, it's important to look at the composition of the body weight, too. BMI can be a useful tool for average people to point out health risks, and it can provide an indication of where your health status currently is. It's also really easy to use, making it quick to assess changes over time.

Rather than comparing yourself to others, I suggest using BMI to compare you to *you*. Is your BMI staying the same? Or does it go up a bit every year? Tracking changes in your BMI can give an indication of whether your weight is headed in the right or wrong direction. You can find BMI calculators easily on the internet or in many health apps for your phone.

Body Fat Percentage

For people wanting to know a bit more information about where they carry more fat or how much they carry, body fat percentage can give a bigger picture. There are many ways to assess body fat, so I'm not going to go into lots of detail here.

Although underwater submersion is the gold standard, it's not easy to do. Skin calipers are typically the best way to assess where you store your fat and identify health risks connected to those areas. This is only accurate based on the competency of the tester (it takes practice to produce reliable results) and can only be used accurately in leaner populations. This makes it challenging to take body fat percentage measurements quickly in a doctor's office. That's why you don't often see studies about body fat percentage in your average population when compared to other measurement tools.

Waist Circumference

Belly fat is connected to disease. That's the visceral fat I mentioned earlier. It's hard to measure the amount of fat inside of you without special equipment, but taking a waist circumference can help. Most credible sources suggest maintaining a waist circumference of less than 102 centimeters for men and less than 88 centimeters for women. Waist circumferences above this are well studied and connected to higher disease risk. I question whether these waist circumferences are a bit generous for most people and should be reduced further.

Regardless of my personal thoughts, this one is easy for you to do in the comfort of your own home. Take a flexible tape measure, wrap it around the smallest part of your waist, and voila—you know your waist circumference. Just make sure you don't cinch the tape measure in tight. It should rest loosely on top of your skin. Keep your fingers out from under it as well!

Getting Diagnosed

Part of accepting a medical condition comes from undergoing the process of getting diagnosed. A diagnosis can come from having specific symptoms, although you may not be at a phase in the disease process where you have started to show or notice symptoms. Beyond using symptoms alone as indicators, you can undergo diagnostic imaging tests such as an X-rays to identify a broken bone or a CT scan to confirm a brain bleed. These tests are specific to each individual case, so I won't expand on them further.

Lab Tests

Lab tests don't always show the full picture, but they will give you an indication of your current health status. Lab testing can be very useful as a baseline diagnostic test to see what's happening under the surface. It can tell you what diseases are starting to develop, because you may not have any symptoms yet.

The downfall of lab testing comes from how the reference interval values are decided. That's the reference range to say if your blood work is too high or too low for a specific marker. Setting these ranges is tricky business! These markers are prone to many variables and should be adjusted for different populations, gender, age, and if the person is healthy or unhealthy.

The problem with setting a reference interval is that there is no *one* way to do this, so each individual lab will set their own standards. The overly simplified version of how they do this is to select a population of at least 120 healthy participants to sample. The trouble begins at this stage because there is absolutely no way to rule out that there is an underlying disease process brewing. It's estimated that 5 percent of the healthy sample population will have results that fall outside of the normal range and will be removed from the sample. That doesn't mean that the other 95 percent remaining are actually healthy.

As we look at the increase in diseases over the past several decades, it would make sense to assume that there is a lot of underlying illness that is not yet diagnosed. We are using participants like this to determine our normal lab values. It is for this reason that I suggest that we lower the reference intervals connected to our chronic diseases.

By the time a person is diagnosed with diabetes, they have already lost between 40 and 50 percent of the function of the beta cells in their pancreas (the ones that help with insulin production.) So why do we wait until you've lost half of your function before we deal with the issue? Since diabetes is costing our health care systems so much, why do we not inform patients much earlier that they are headed down the path to diabetes?

If you were aware of the consequences much earlier in the process, you'd have time to make lifestyle changes that could delay or prevent the onset of diabetes, ultimately saving thousands of dollars in treatment down the line. Multiply this number by the population at risk for diabetes, and we could be saving billions of dollars worldwide. Think of how much of a difference that money could make if put to other uses!

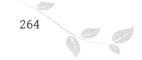

Lab tests are not irrelevant, nor do I mean to imply that they are. What I do suggest is that we use lab tests to identify small changes in your blood work over time so that we can give you the information much sooner than is currently being done. Just because your lab work is *normal* doesn't mean that's an ideal scenario. Take charge of your own health, and if you see lab results such as your blood sugar trending on the high end of *normal,* know that it's time to make some lifestyle changes to dial it back.

Here Comes the Diagnosis

You've now been diagnosed with a disease based on a combination of your lab testing, diagnostic imaging, and symptoms. Now what?

While it's not great news that you aren't well, it's good that you now have knowledge and can do something about it. To take things one step further, you should look into the cause of your condition. Are you sick because you eat too many carbohydrate-rich foods? Or perhaps because you are inactive? Maybe your stress level is through the roof and you don't get enough sleep.

It's important to have respect for a well-supported clinical diagnosis, even if you don't believe it to be true. Feel free to get a second opinion—that will help to ensure you are receiving correct information. What worries me is when people are in denial and refuse to follow through on a diagnosis. I've worked with clients who have told me that they don't believe they have diabetes or high blood pressure because they don't feel sick.

Some people have blood sugar levels so high that they should go to the hospital immediately, yet they feel no different than when their sugars are in a normal range. Or they stop taking their hypertensive medication because their recent blood pressures have all been in the normal range. It was in the normal range because the medication is doing its job.

This sounds mean, but it honestly doesn't matter what you think. If you have a medical condition, then you can't make it go away by ignoring it. You can, however, improve your odds by changing how you apply different lifestyle habits.

Your body is a lean, mean healing machine. It knows how to heal itself; you just need to give it a chance to heal. When you cut your hand or scrape your knee, it heals over time. By setting the right conditions through your lifestyle, you can *heal* chronic diseases. While you may not *technically* be able to heal a disease or chronic condition, you can effectively manage it through lifestyle choices. This makes it appear as though you have healed or cured your medical condition. At the minimum, you can decrease the severity of your symptoms or improve your quality of life. You can't just *heal* a medical condition by carrying on with the same habits that got you there. You have to set up the right conditions for your body to heal itself.

Focus on Your Health

Wherever you focus, that is where your attention goes. In some ways, we focus too much on our health, while in other ways, we focus too little. I absolutely believe that we should focus on the big picture and really look at all the things that we could be doing to positively impact our health. But sometimes, we are absolutely clueless about what's really happening in our bodies.

Half the time, you aren't even aware of how crappy you feel because you have become so accustomed to feeling like garbage that it becomes your new normal. Jennifer came to see me for weight loss and complained of low energy. She begged me to give her the motivation to lose weight. Jennifer had struggled to stick with previous weight loss attempts. After teaching her many of the tips I've shared with you, she was able to lose a few pounds. That inspired her to lose a few more and created some forward momentum.

The more weight Jennifer lost, the more energy she reported having. Just think of how much more energy you could have if I didn't make you carry around a sack of potatoes every day! That's exactly what weight loss is doing. Helping to put down that sack of potatoes so your body can rest and recover. Energy goes up as a result. Jennifer didn't even realize how sluggish she was until she started to feel better. She created a new normal.

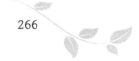

On the flip side, you can focus too much on medical conditions. You can get so caught up in your disease process that you take on the persona of the disease. *I am a diabetic. I am a cancer patient. I'm an amputee.* Yes, you might have those conditions, but they do not define you. You are a man and father who happens to have diabetes. You are a successful CEO and triathlete who has been diagnosed with cancer. Or you are a war hero who fought for your country and had a leg amputation. You are so much more than just a disease. It's not *your cancer*; you don't own it. It's *the* cancer in your breast. Change your language, and you'll be surprised at how you can separate yourself from the disease.

You can also focus so much on a medical condition that you pretty much walk around with blinders on, only noticing things pertaining to that disease. In the digestion chapter, I spoke about how you suddenly notice red cars after you buy one yourself. Similar to how you can focus too much on your digestion, you can do the same with other medical conditions. You become hyper-vigilant, and you notice *everything*. Even things you aren't supposed to notice.

I had surgery on both of my shins to address a chronic condition that was causing me excruciating pain. Through my recovery process, I ended up getting severe nerve pain in one leg. The nerves had become hyper-vigilant and were fired up like crazy. They told me *everything* that was happening to them! I could barely touch my own leg, and the water drops when taking a shower felt like daggers slicing into my skin. It was absolutely no fun at all. This nerve pain was almost worse than the pain I had before, and I knew I couldn't live with it for the rest of my life. So I aggressively sought out other perspectives on how to treat it.

Your nervous system, like mine, can get cranked up and fire off a ton of messages telling you that you have pain, when in fact, your body has actually healed. This is a real phenomenon and happens to people all the time. Your body is healed—your nerves are just sending your brain a different message. You are not crazy, I promise! It's in these situations that you need to turn attention away from your condition. I'll share what helped me get through this in Chapter Twenty-Two: Pain.

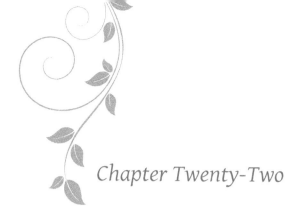

Chapter Twenty-Two

Pain

I included a section on pain in Chapter Thirteen: Deepening Your Knowledge to specifically talk about how to exercise while in pain. This chapter focuses on other strategies to help manage pain. The cost of pain on society has huge implications not only on health care but on productivity, absenteeism, presenteeism, quality of life, and the economy as a whole. In the United Kingdom, the annual cost of back pain alone was estimated to be £1 billion, with around £69 million being spent on primary care management of chronic pain conditions. Australia estimates 9.9 million work days lost annually due to pain. Chronic pain affects as high as 60 percent of the world's population or more, depending on the evaluation methods used. It's no wonder that pain is costing our health care systems so much!

Some common predictors for having pain include having a low level of education, being under psychological distress, or having other comorbidities. By not treating pain—or treating it ineffectively—complications arise. There can be an increase in mental symptoms such as depression or anxiety from social isolation and loss of mobility. Health care utilization also goes up with increased pain, resulting in higher treatment costs.

Many patients don't complain about their pain because they don't want to be a burden or a nuisance to their medical team. They might be worried about the consequences of gaining an injury or pain diagnosis, especially in countries where patients incur the costs for hospitalization, drugs, or other treatment options. There's also a misconception that pain is a normal part of aging, which it is not.

Chronic Pain vs. Acute Pain

There are two key types of pain: acute and chronic. Acute pain is of a sudden onset and usually resolves within a few days to months. Acute pain generally comes from some type of injury or illness that can be resolved with or without treatment. Chronic pain typically lasts longer than six months and may or may not originate from acute pain. Chronic pain can be more debilitating and in some cases receives little to no benefit from treatment. This is the type of pain that costs our health care systems billions of dollars annually.

What is Pain?

So, what does this mysterious thing called chronic pain look like? How do you know if someone is in pain? Unfortunately, chronic pain has a bad stigma because it's difficult to identify. You can't tell that someone's pain just by looking at them. In nursing school, I learned, "pain is what you say it is." You might have severe pain and look perfectly normal. That doesn't mean that you aren't experiencing those symptoms.

Not all pain can be cured. In these cases, you'll need to learn ways to live with pain and still have a happy, balanced life. That's not to minimize the fact that you have pain but rather, to develop a new expectation for what's realistic *now*.

Pain can affect any area of your body, including bones, muscles, joints, nerves, or organs. It can range in severity from sharp, jagged, burning, or

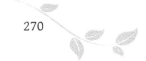

stabbing to gnawing, grating, throbbing, pounding, dull, or aching. Pain can cause additional symptoms such as numbness, tingling, tightness, swelling, or a pulling sensation, depending on the cause. Pain causes a significant impact on physical, psychological, and sociological functioning due to the way that it intertwines itself with every aspect of your life.

Pain-Depression Spiral

As I'm sure you're starting to understand, pain is a complex interaction between many factors. Typically, it starts out fairly benign; you develop pain.

Most people can tolerate pain for the short term; it's when the pain continues or is not managed that problems start to arise. With pain, we recommend rest and passive coping strategies to help your body heal. As the pain persists, you'll experience a limitation on the amount of activity you can participate in without increasing or exacerbating the pain. This decrease in activity leads to increased tightness and stiffness, and if left too long, can lead to weak or tight muscles and a decline in fitness.

Pain

↓

Limited Activity

↓

Tightness/Stiffness

↓

Withdrawal

↓

Anxiety, Depression, Anger

The next phase results in withdrawal from social activities due to the pain or inability to participate in a given activity. Social isolation contributes to a decrease in mood and self-esteem, a change in sleep habits, weight gain or loss, and strain on relationships. These frustrations compound and can lead to feelings of anger, depression, and anxiety.

You are depressed, so you don't do things, so you tighten up from lack of movement, so you have less mobility, so you withdraw more and your pain gets worse . . . and on and on and on.

To complicate this spiral even further, your nervous system can get stuck in overdrive. It can be so turned on that it keeps firing off messages that you have pain, even long after your original injury has healed. (That's what happened to me.) There is much more research coming out now about how to down-regulate those hormones to stop producing pain signals. I anticipate much more information in the next several years helping to manage chronic pain much more effectively than current medications can.

Passive Coping

This type of coping is very inactive. It's a quick fix, where you don't have to participate very much. You take a pill or use an ice/heat pack. You get a procedure done to fix your problem. You show up for some type of hands-on therapy where someone else does the work on you. This can range from ultrasound, TENS, massage, or acupuncture to some types of physiotherapy. Passive coping strategies are great for acute pain or chronic pain in its early stages. It seems to be a more common option today, especially if you want to be *fixed* by someone else. Passive coping is only so effective; sometimes you need to do more.

Active Coping

This form of coping requires you to be an active participant in dealing with your concerns. You have to put in some work or effort to take control of your pain. The focus of active coping can help you to move away from a pain-centered life through a focus on education as well as exploring other options for medical and alternative treatments.

Active coping comes down to using self-management skills that allow you to pace yourself and step away from the pain-depression spiral. It does not necessarily mean that you will become pain-free. Active coping techniques help you to implement relaxation, exercise and pacing strategies to help you increase your activity level. This helps to increase your

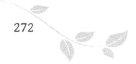

strength, flexibility, and fitness, which positively impact your mood and ability to be social.

Part of stepping out of the pain-depression spiral active process involves reprogramming your brain. Once your nervous system gets amped up, you'll need to use other ways to dial it back down. Tara Brach, a PhD level Psychologist describes RAIN, a mindfulness-based meditation to help get through stressful or painful times. Ronald Siegel, PsyD, takes this one step further and directly applies this concept to pain. By recognizing that your pain changes from minute to minute, and understanding that you are not your pain, you will gain more control over your life. These tools, put together from both of these well-educated professionals, helped me to not only deal with nerve pain but to heal it without the use of medication.

While I was working on the psychology side of desensitizing my nerves, I had to give my body a chance to do the same. At first, all I had to do was lay a hand lightly on my legs. Sounds simple, but it hurt so badly. I had to teach my body that it was safe when confronted by light touch. Over time, I was able to gradually increase pressure and change the sensation by tapping or rubbing the skin.

Once I was no longer getting benefit from that, I had to step it up a notch. That's where my partner came in. He started just with a simple touch, but I felt like my pain got worse when he did it. That's because the touch was unpredictable. It was out of *my* control, and I couldn't anticipate what was going to happen. As I tolerated his touch more, he was able to follow the same progression that I had done.

This effort still hadn't taken care of all of my nerve pain, and a beach vacation was rapidly approaching. I reluctantly went on holidays, concerned about my walking endurance and pain level when anything unpredictable happened to my legs. It was the best thing that I could have done! Standing on the edge of the ocean with the warm water lapping up on my legs felt like little knives cutting into me. I hated it. (How is that the best thing I could have done? Keep reading!)

Knowing that I was safe and wasn't harming my body by doing this (it was actually encouraged by my doctor), I was able to slowly relax and

273

tolerate the water. By the end of the week, the water no longer caused the same pain it had on the first day. I went home and was able to continue to expose my legs to new movements and new sensations and eventually was able to heal my nerve pain. It took months of effort every day but was well worth it in the end. I would never have put in that much effort without the encouragement and support I was given.

Again, not all pain can be healed, but I suspect that most people can make a significant improvement to their pain levels with a little persistence. Along the way, you'll want to plan for flare-ups. They will happen, and that's a normal part of the recovery process. It's not something you did wrong.

Acknowledging that you are having a flare-up will take the blame away from you. It diffuses the emotional charge that comes with it. Use a combination of passive and active coping strategies to get you through the flare and back on track. If flare-ups happen too often, you may need to reassess your rehabilitation plan and slow things down a bit so you aren't constantly playing catch-up.

Pillar 7: Lifestyle Factors

"Because the biological mechanisms that affect our health and well-being are so dynamic, when people change their diet and lifestyle, they usually feel so much better, so quickly; it reframes the reason for changing from fear of dying to joy of living. Also, the support that patients give each other is a powerful motivator."

—DEAN ORNISH

"Your genetics load the gun. Your lifestyle pulls the trigger."

—MEHMET OZ (DR. OZ)

"When I work, a lot of times I have to lose weight, and I do that, but in my regular life I was not eating right, and I was not getting enough exercise. But by the nature of my diet and that lifestyle—boom! The end result was high blood sugars that reach the levels where it becomes type two diabetes. I share that with a gajillion other people."

—TOM HANKS

Chapter Twenty-Three

What Are Your Lifestyle Factors?

*Y*our lifestyle factors are pretty much everything else that I haven't talked about in this book so far. The only thing that's consistent about lifestyle factors is the inconsistency between them. They are all the components that make you special and unique—the things that make your situation different from everyone else's. Not everyone has the same lifestyle factors, nor do they occur at the same time as you or in the same way. Your lifestyle factors are unique to you and in the way that they impact you, similar to the epigenetic factors.

Lifestyle factors interact with all the other components of your health. They are that drop of water in your bucket that makes it overflow. Sometimes, they are the giant tidal wave that rocks your world or makes your table collapse. Each lifestyle factor on its own is not necessarily that problematic, but they will stress any weakness or imbalance you have in other areas.

Due to the unique nature of each lifestyle factor and how it positively or negatively impacts you, I've chosen to keep this chapter short and sweet. Each concept could easily be expanded into a chapter of its own, but I'll keep things to a minimum. Have a read through each concept and take note of how these factors may be influencing your overall health. How can you take some of the weight off of your table by addressing these simple yet important factors?

Regular Body Maintenance

This concept comes down to the ways that you look after your own body. Just like a car, there's some regular maintenance to do. You need to perform oil changes, keep it filled up with gas and washer fluid, and occasionally take your car to the car wash to prevent it from developing rust. In the same way, you need to do basic hygiene and routine maintenance for your health.

You can start by checking your user manual and seeing how often you are due for your next scheduled maintenance. All right, you don't really have a user manual, but there are suggestions by health care professionals on how often you should be seeing them. You should go for a check-up with your physician, dentist, and optometrist or ophthalmologist at least annually. These regular checkups are the diagnostic assessments to see if you have a headlight that's burnt out or if your tire pressure is a bit low. Your car can still run if these things are out of whack, but you aren't operating at the best of your abilities. By detecting health issues when they are small, through routine maintenance, it'll save you from having to replace your transmission prematurely.

With age, it's also important to screen for your hearing. It is normal to have a decline in hearing certain pitches with age, but it's vitally important to maintain a normal level of hearing. Not only does poor hearing create social isolation, it actually causes brain cells to die off because they are no longer being stimulated by sound waves. To prevent this permanent loss of brain cells, get a hearing aid as early as possible and use it regularly.

Smaller hygiene tasks that you perform regularly can have a significant impact on your health. Tanner was shocked by how much lower his blood sugar numbers were after a getting a dental cleaning. Routine dental checks can help to identify bacterial buildup that may be negatively affecting your blood sugar. Brushing and flossing your teeth can have a

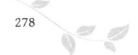

significant impact on keeping these bacteria at bay. So when you listen to your dental hygienist's recommendation to brush and floss daily, it may positively impact more than just the health of your mouth.

Showering regularly also falls into this same category, removing bacteria, yeast, and fungus that may get tucked away into those lovely, moist crevices of your body. In normal conditions, your immune system keeps these under control, but it can sometimes get out of balance and cause skin infections. How good are you at regular body maintenance? What can you do to improve this area?

Safety

Here come the fun police! It's not about taking away all of your fun; it's just about making sure that you do things in a safe and controlled manner. Some people participate in risky behaviors much more often than others who are very risk averse. Where do you sit in this spectrum? Some people are willing to jump out of airplanes with a tiny piece of fabric strapped to their backs that's supposed to prevent them from crashing into the earth. Sometimes, the parachute works, while other times, catastrophe strikes, and it's all over in a matter of seconds. When you make decisions to partake in risky activities, you have to be willing to accept the harsh consequences.

It doesn't have to be such a dramatic example, either. I've seen people who have just had bad luck in normal, everyday situations. I met a patient who became quadriplegic from falling the wrong way when sitting on a paint bucket. Or a successful businessman who died of complications after hitting his head on the ice when he was curling.

Sometimes, bad stuff happens to good people. Not that we need to cover ourselves in bubble wrap just to get through a day. It's about assessing the probability of something happening to us. It's about identifying what the potential risks or hazards are in your chosen activity and determining if the risk is worth the reward. If you're young and single, your risk adversity might be greater than that of a new mother. Maybe not!

Some other ways for you to reduce your risk are by regularly using safety equipment such as helmets and seatbelts. They are proven to reduce the chance of injury or death when used correctly. It's also wise to practice safe sex and protect yourself with appropriate contraceptive devices or through abstinence. Unwanted pregnancies and sexually transmitted infections are largely preventable. Lastly, protect your skin from damaging UV rays by using the correct type of sunscreen and clothing options or by staying out of the sun when UV ratings are high.

Busyness

Hurry up, you need to get more done! That seems to be the mantra of modern society. Do more. Be more. Produce more. We are driven to think that being busy is a badge of honor. But being busy doesn't always produce results. In fact, it appears to do the opposite.

To an extent, you need to put in more hours to get more stuff done, but there's a fine balance before productivity starts to decline. How you manage your time will often dictate how effective you are in other aspects of your life. Ever notice when you slow down and take a break that you can get more done in far less time? Running around like a chicken with your head cut off all the time isn't helping you get more done. It's holding you back.

Learn to delegate tasks to family members or hire out someone to help so that you aren't doing everything yourself. I'm a bit of a control freak and like to have my hand in pretty much everything, so this part is hard for me. What I've noticed is that the more I let go of things, the more productive I can be in other areas of my life. So ask for help and support to lighten your load.

If you have kids, you'll want them to grow up to be fully functioning adults one day, right? So help them learn those essential skills like cooking, laundry, and cleaning from an early age. Your kids shouldn't become your slaves, but I firmly believe that they should partake in the running of a household with increasing responsibility, as they get older.

Do the things that are most important to you first. Be just a wee bit selfish for once and take care of your own needs before everyone else's. My female clients tend to struggle with this more than my male clients, likely because of the mothering role that can be expected of us.

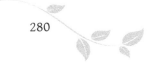

Sometimes, your time can be dictated for you, as in the case of shift work or other jobs where you work set hours. It can be challenging to manage your work schedule when the hours don't match up with your ideal life. Recognize that rotating hours or shifts that are during evening or night hours will put a larger strain on your health. If you fall into this category, you'll need to be extra diligent about balancing the other factors in your table of health.

Balance

On top of being busy, it comes down to how you balance everything that's thrown your way. I touched on this in Pillar 4: Mental Health, but it's so important that I'm going to include more about it.

Balance doesn't mean that *everything* needs to get done 100 percent all the time. In fact, sometimes balance involves making a conscious choice to **not** do something, even if you really want to. It comes down to deciding what's really realistic and what's not. You aren't Superwoman or Superman, and you can't be all things to all people.

Riley has always been high-drive and super ambitious. She went directly from her undergraduate degree into medical school and had plans to pursue a surgical residency. During her undergraduate degree, she found that running was a great stress relief for her. So she started doing it more and more. Eventually, her path led to running marathons, qualifying for the Boston Marathon. She turned to triathlons for additional cross training and eventually committed herself to doing Ironman.

Riley is very health conscious and concerned about ethics, so she eats a strict vegetarian diet, bordering on being vegan. Only she's not a great vegetarian. She eats lots of processed food—candy and granola bars are the staple of her diet. After all, she's a busy med student on weird shift rotations and doesn't have much time to cook. A good meal is a salad with a bit of cheese and nuts on top for protein.

What Riley doesn't understand is why she's always injured. It's been multiple stress fractures and chronic muscle strains that keep holding her back. Her body is yelling at her to stop, but she hasn't gotten the message yet. Riley's missed qualifying for the coveted Kona Ironman a few times by only a few minutes each time. She works hard, trains hard, and deserves to qualify. What Riley really needs is more balance in her life.

Remember that concept of going slow to go fast? By taking the time to rest and get more than a few hours of sleep at a time, Riley will allow her aching muscles and bones to heal. Training less often will enhance muscle recovery, making her stronger. Focusing on balancing her nutrition by ensuring she's getting the proper balance of amino acids and cutting out the inflammatory, sugary foods will likely give her the sustained energy needed to finally make the qualifying time for Kona.

While doing Kona Ironman may not be your cup of tea, what is that big goal that you keep working towards? Where do you keep getting stuck? If you've been working harder and harder at it with no results, it may be time to take a step back and do less. Sometimes, less is more! Or sometimes, it's shifting the balance of where your focus goes. Maybe you've been in pursuit of exercise for so long you've lost balance in the other key aspects of your health. Take a good look at your overall life balance and see what needs to be adjusted.

Environmental

I'm talking about all the different environments and environmental factors that have an impact on you. Your daily environment has a significant impact on your health, as that's where you spend the majority of your time. If you live or work in an environment with toxins, your body will have to work that much harder to detoxify your system. Sometimes, that toxic load is too much for your body to bear and you end up getting sick. Do what you can to reduce your environmental toxic load by using personal protective equipment in work environments and by reducing chemicals and plastics in your home environment.

Your social determinants of health will also play a role in the way you are treated and what opportunities are available to you. These factors include race, gender, disability, education, income, employment, access to health care, and childhood development. Many of the impacts to your health are tied to your education and the ability to access affordable housing. Without safe and affordable housing, it's nearly impossible

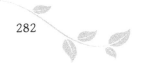

WHAT ARE YOUR LIFESTYLE FACTORS?

to maintain stable employment or to prepare healthy meals. Everyone should have the opportunity to earn a living wage; however, that's far from happening in many countries. If we want to truly make a difference to the burden on health care systems, addressing housing costs and creating a true living wage would make a significant impact.

Other invisible barriers (or sometimes visible barriers) to health come from race, culture, and gender. In some countries, these determinants have more of a significant impact on health than in other countries. It can even vary depending on what part of a country you live in. It's often minority populations, females, and *different* genders that get stigmatized and lose access to services. Just because someone defines their gender differently than you does not mean that they should be denied access to the same opportunities. Yet that's exactly what happens all around the world. In other countries, being born a woman can be a death sentence. The economic and political climate you grow up in will dramatically affect how your determinants of health are impacted.

Nature

The environment you choose to surround yourself with on a regular basis may or may not include being out in nature. You don't have to rush out and go for a polar bear swim (naked in ice-cold water) or get covered in mud to get the benefits of nature. Being in nature can include getting some sunshine on your bare skin, fresh air on your face, or soil underneath your bare feet. It doesn't have to mean a long drive out to the wilderness, although if that's your thing, I highly encourage it!

Being in nature helps to restore balance and give you a sense of being grounded. I know that after a day in the mountains or on a beach, I feel all *zen*. Connecting with nature can help put life in perspective and make your problems seem much more bearable. I used to love running without music because then I was able to sort out all those busy thoughts inside my head. I came back feeling clear-headed. I'm not currently running, but I still use this approach with other activities like hiking or cross-country skiing.

But what if you aren't a big tree hugger? What if you'd prefer to be indoors? Take your indoor hobby outside! Bring your book or laptop outside and sit in the sun for at least a few minutes without sun protection. Ideally, you'll do this when the UV rating is lower and not at the peak of the day, to prevent skin damage. You do, however, want to get a few minutes of sun exposure to pump up your vitamin D stores to help improve your mood. The goal is not to turn your skin into fruit leather! If you live somewhere colder, like me, this isn't possible all year round. So dress for the weather and go for a walk instead.

When you are outside, try to head somewhere where there are trees or large amounts of grasses and plants. If it's warm enough to take off your shoes and walk on the earth, do this daily for the grounding effects. Walking on natural surfaces like grass, sand, or dirt will give you a deeper connection to the earth than the paved patio in your backyard. Remember to breathe deeply and slowly while in nature to get lots of fresh, clean air into your body.

Family

Family responsibilities can be incredibly joyous and fulfilling, but they can also take a toll on your health. Anyone who puts in additional time taking care of a young family will understand what I mean. Perhaps you've got young children and need to manage the childcare responsibilities. If you're up all night with a newborn or a fussy toddler, then it's hard to have enough energy to get anything done the next day, let alone excel at healthy habits.

The pressure to have children may be high. Not every couple can have kids, and not every couple wants kids. Some couples can't even agree on their plans together. When these pressures are high—and in contrast to your personal beliefs—you'll experience additional stress. For some, that stress comes from wanting a deeper connection with someone and being unable to find a suitable partner.

Maybe you have a family member with special needs who requires personal care beyond your typical relationship. Being a caregiver can be difficult and thankless work. You're possibly in a caregiver role for your aging parents. For some people, this adds value to their day while others

feel overwhelmed and burdened by their parents' unrealistic expectations for support.

Even in your household, demanding partners or pets can eat up your time or add stress (on top of all the love they bring). It's incredibly hard to make the decision to euthanize an aging pet or to lose a pet to natural causes. Not unlike the death of a family member, you can undergo a similar grieving process. And the stress associated with the death of a family member—especially children—can be astronomical.

Vaginal Birth

At this point, it's far too late to change how *you* were born, so that's a moot point. You can, however, influence the type of birth your future children may have. The research supporting the benefits of having a vaginal birth is astounding. There's absolutely no reason why you shouldn't opt for this as your first option unless you've been told by your doctor that you *need* to have a delivery by cesarean section.

To be clear, if you or someone you know falls into this category, no harm, no foul—that's out of your control, and I certainly won't hold it against you. The first priority is to keep mom and baby safe, and sometimes, that does mean turning to surgical options.

But if you are opting for an elective cesarean section just because you don't want to push a baby out, I'd like to encourage you to change your mind. (Full disclosure, I have not had any children at this point and have no idea what it's like to push a watermelon out of my tiny vagina. However, if I did have kids, I'd opt for a natural birth if possible.) By having a vaginal delivery, the baby gets mucus squeezed out of their body from the delivery process, helping to reduce respiratory symptoms. Babies are also typically able to start breastfeeding sooner after a vaginal delivery than a cesarean section delivery.

Through a vaginal delivery, your baby will be inoculated with bacteria from the birth canal, helping to build a more robust immune system, and may have lower risk of obesity, allergies, and asthma. In fact, new research is coming out suggesting that babies born from cesarean births should be inoculated with the good bacteria from mom's vagina. There are no long-term studies on this protocol, but short-term studies seem promising. If possible, consider a vaginal birth as the first option to providing your baby with a solid foundation for their health.

Lifestyle Habits

Beyond the other lifestyle factors, you also make personal choices about your lifestyle habits. They overlap with other key pillars of health but deserve to be mentioned again here. Do you participate in addictive behaviors such as smoking, drinking, or drug use? These substances all affect the way that you think and act and will have influence over your other health decisions.

The importance of social connections is well cited in the literature for supporting changes in lifestyle habits. Having regular interactions with other people with the same goals will increase your chance of success. Set your intention for better health and surround yourself with others who can support you along your journey.

Whether or not you are open to changing your routine or habits will determine your ability to stick to change. Making a change to appease a health care practitioner or a nagging family member doesn't usually create a long-term, sustainable change. You have to be interested and willing to partake in your own health.

Putting It All Together: Final Thoughts

"Modern disease is a result of a mismatch of our genetic makeup and our lifestyle."

—STANLEY BOYD EATON, AUTHOR OF
THE PALEOLITHIC PRESCRIPTION

"Follow your dreams, work hard, practice, and persevere. Make sure you eat a variety of foods, get plenty of exercise, and maintain a healthy lifestyle."

—SASHA COHEN

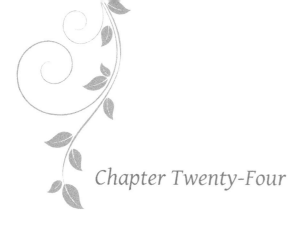

Chapter Twenty-Four

Integrating Your
New Knowledge

*Y*ou've just learned a lot of new information, or perhaps you've gotten a new perspective on things that you already knew. This book is not about examining every single little detail of each topic, or it would be way too long. I've given you enough information so that you don't have to read several different books before you can start making changes.

The bigger question is, what are you going to do with this new information? There's a difference between learning new information and then actually implementing the knowledge you just learned. Stop reading book after book and getting frustrated about not seeing the results they promise. It's the *changes* that you make based on that knowledge that are going to get you somewhere.

Where Does Your Information Come From?

This book would not be complete without a warning: Be careful about where you find your health information.

I recently watched a documentary on food, and it made me so mad that I had to turn it off. It was full of blatantly incorrect information. The problem is, most people don't know that!

While documentaries are fantastic for evoking emotions and getting you excited to join a cause, they aren't always credible. The same is true for media stories. So when you are choosing information for making key lifestyle changes, really think about who you are getting your information from. Is it a close friend or family member? What's their education? Where did they learn the information? If it came from a television show, a magazine, or a short blog post, it may not be fully credible. It may have some element of truth, but it may have been twisted into a sensationalized media story.

I think it's also important to look at the health habits of the person giving you the advice. Do they always seem to be on a diet? Or following the newest fitness fad? This person may be an early adopter of new fads without really finding out what research the activity is based on. Is your new health mentor giving you tips to be healthy when they aren't really healthy themselves? The person you take lifestyle advice from should be willing to walk the walk and practice what they preach.

What if You Don't Agree with Everything in This Book?

There's a (really good) chance that you aren't going to agree with everything I've written in this book. In fact, you might even believe that something I've shared is false based on your unique background or conflicting information you've read elsewhere. And that's okay. Let it go. If something doesn't resonate with you, let it be. But I do challenge you to find some other way to continue to improve each and every pillar of your health in some way.

It's also important to recognize that information is always changing, especially regarding health topics. Rather than judging me, give me the right to update this book and change my mind when new information becomes available. That will help me to continue producing quality information based on current research to help you on your journey.

By no means do I have it all figured out. Far from it! The more I learn, the more I realize I don't know. So, like me, keep learning and keep experimenting to find what works for you. If it doesn't give you ideal results, discard it and try again.

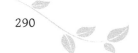

Starting New Lifestyle Habits

I've seen this saying phrased in so many different ways: "If you keep doing the things you have been doing, you'll keep getting the same results that you have been getting." This may be a good thing, or it may be a bad thing depending on your happiness with your current health.

The problem with health-related habits is that the negative impact from your choices doesn't usually rear its ugly head until months or years later. Chronic diseases typically develop slowly over time through a combination of your genetic programming and your lifestyle factors. How did you get diabetes? Where did those extra thirty pounds come from? It feels like they just snuck up on you. But they've actually been brewing in the background for years.

Since you've likely had your current habits for a long time, it's going to take some time to change them as well. If you've had an unhealthy habit for most of your life, it's likely going to take more than the standard twenty-one days to change it. Keep at it and know that you will make mistakes along the way. Things will not be perfect or go smoothly the first few times.

New Year's is the time when the greatest number of people resolve to change their lifestyle habits. Many people start with goals that are too ambitious, end up burning out about a month or two later, and then repeat the same pattern again the next year. Developing long-term lifestyle habits takes time and should be done in a progressive fashion to achieve lasting results.

If you want to lose fifty pounds and set out to accomplish that goal by never touching another desert again, you'd be setting yourself up for failure. Not to say that someone with extremely high willpower and strong motivation to be successful couldn't achieve that goal—perhaps someone could. But many people make so many changes so abruptly that they feel deprived and end up binging on an entire cake. A better way to accomplish that same goal would be to make one or two dietary changes each month so that you have time to adapt to a new way of eating without the same feelings of deprivation.

It is impossible to change your body overnight. It took several years to get that belly or to grow those love handles. It will take a while to get them to disappear, too. You are bombarded by media ads and trendy diets showing you quick-fix solutions for weight loss and body transformation. Sadly, quick fixes don't produce lasting results. Keep focused on the slow and steady approach to making longer-lasting changes.

Now, if you're concerned about making changes too slowly, think about the lasting impact of those changes. Imagine if you integrated a new healthy habit every day for only five minutes. Think about how much time that would add up to over the course of the next twenty years of your life. That works out to 608 hours! You could be an entirely new person if you devoted 608 hours to healthy habits. Changing your eating or exercise habits may take up to a year but will be well worth it in the end. Your new behavior becomes your new normal over time.

This is a great time to consider how your current habits compare to other people. What are the habits of healthy people? There are lots of existing books on this topic, but the key takeaway is that they *actually do* the things that make them—and keep them—healthy. Sounds pretty achievable, right?

Healthy people *make* time to prepare meals, work out, have downtime, sleep, and do things that recharge their batteries. Think of the healthiest person you know. What do they do differently than you? What can you learn from their habits? Keep these thoughts in mind as you start designing your healthy future.

I think back to when I first started really taking care of my health, I felt completely overwhelmed. There were so many things to do. And so many things to think about. I ended up being very frustrated and felt quite deprived because I no longer fit in with my social circle. Over the years, I've learned to pace myself and only take on one or two new things at a time.

I didn't develop my current lifestyle overnight. It took me years to learn the skills and habits I have now. Keep that in perspective if you try to compare yourself with others! Start with small, manageable chunks and keep building on them over time. You'll get there eventually!

Imagine Your Future

This is your chance to imagine what your new healthy lifestyle looks like. At this point, you don't have to know how to do it, only where you want to go and why you want it. You can imagine any future for yourself as long as it's in the realm of possibility. I don't want you to set yourself up for failure by imagining a future that isn't physically possible. If you have a completely severed spinal cord and will never be able to walk again, you'd be disappointed if your exercise goal was to run a marathon. A more realistic goal would be to race the marathon in a sport wheelchair.

I want you to push yourself out of your current comfort zone and ask more of yourself than you have in the past. Know that you can achieve most goals with sheer determination and hard work. Here are a few questions to ask yourself to set some direction for your future:

▷ What factors about having a new, healthy lifestyle are important to you?
▷ What would you lose by changing your current lifestyle habits?
▷ What would you gain by changing your current lifestyle habits?
▷ What is holding you back from making changes?
▷ Who would this change affect or impact? How?
▷ What would your ideal and realistic body look like?
▷ How would you feel in your body with your new lifestyle habits?
▷ What activities do you like to do? Or enjoyed doing in the past?
▷ What have you always wanted to try but were too afraid to do—or didn't know how?

Answering these questions will help you clearly envision a new, healthy future. It's very important at this point to understand *why* you are making changes. The more authentic these reasons are, the more success you will have in achieving your goals. Find the reasons that really tug on your heartstrings. They will resonate with you and keep you on track much longer than superficial reasons. Now that you have a clear vision of where you want to go, we can move on to identifying the steps you'll need to take to get you there.

Identifying Your Starting Point

It's easy to postpone making changes to your lifestyle for numerous different reasons. The best time to start making changes is right now. They don't even have to be big changes. You'll want to know where you are starting from so that you can have a way to track your progress. Here are a few questions for you to think about to determine your current starting point. Answer each of them as you go through and record your answers so that you can look back to see where you started from.

Sleep
- How much sleep do you actually get each night?
- What's the quality of your sleep?
- Do you snore or wake up feeling tired?
- Do you take naps?

Nutrition
- How much food are you eating?
- What is the quality of the food you eat?
- What are your kitchen cupboards filled with?

Exercise
- What is your daily activity level?
- Do you exercise?
- What is your current level of fitness?
- What does your body look like right now? (Include your height, weight, waist circumference, blood pressure, and any other measurements if possible.)

Mental Health
- How much time do you spend watching TV or on the computer?
- Who does all the work around the house?
- What is your self-talk like? (I'm too fat, I'm too tired.)
- What stressors do you have in your life right now? (Good and bad.)

Digestion
- How often do you have bowel movements?
- How hard to you have to work to have a bowel movement?
- Do you have symptoms of gas, bloating, diarrhea, or constipation?
- How often do these occur?

Medical Conditions
- Do you have a diagnosed illness, injury, or medical condition?
- Do you go for annual checkups with your doctor, dentist, and eye doctor?
- How do you handle concerns as they arise?
- Do you have a list of all of your medications, supplements, and herbal remedies?

Lifestyle Factors
- How is your current energy level? Does it fluctuate during the day? Is it constant?
- What unhealthy choices do you make on a daily basis that affect your health? (e.g., smoking, foods, exercise, taking the stairs instead of the elevator, toxic work environment.)
- Is this current lifestyle helping you to be the fit, healthy, active person you want to be?

Great job! Sometimes, it's hard to be honest with yourself and really look at the picture with both eyes wide open. You've taken the first step to acknowledging where you are right now. You may have just discovered some new things about yourself that you never really realized before. Or perhaps you've increased your awareness of unhealthy habits you've had for years. Either way, now you have a greater awareness of where you stand.

Take a look through your answers and see if there are one or two areas that are more out of balance than the others. Plan to start working on these first. If you think *all* of your areas are out of balance, that's okay too. Pick the top two that you think will make the biggest impact on your health. Remember these areas for the next step.

To get you on the road to success, I've included a free 30-day Quick Start Guide. You'll get a free downloadable PDF guide that walks you through a plan of how to rebalance each of your key pillars of health. Check it out at: www.yourlifestylestrategy.com/bookbonus

Set Your Goals

You'll want to create some tangible goals to help you work towards the ideal future you've just spent some time designing. Since you can't do everything at once, I'm going to help you build a master plan and then break it up into manageable pieces.

Start out by identifying five things you can do for each pillar of health to get you closer to your greater vision of health. There will be some new habits that you will need to start doing and current habits that you may need to stop doing. To me, it doesn't matter which column they fall in as long as you have five new strategies for each pillar of health.

GOAL-SETTING MATRIX		
	What will you start doing?	What will you stop doing?
Sleep		
Nutrition		
Exercise		
Mental Health		
Digestion		
Medical Conditions		
Lifestyle Factors		

Now that you have a big list of habits to change, you'll need to make that more manageable. Remember your top two pillars that were most out of balance? That's where I want you to start.

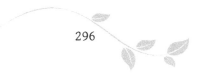

I like overlapping a few different aspects of health so that you don't get overwhelmed by doing too many new things at once. Let's pretend that for you, they are nutrition and sleep. Pick one or two healthy habits for nutrition and sleep that you can start doing today. You could start by making your room as dark as possible at night and having protein every morning at breakfast. Although you're starting two new habits at once, they don't create too much change in any one aspect of your life. Once your room is set up for better sleep, it doesn't take much work to maintain it (other than keeping it clean!). Then you can move on to another habit for sleep hygiene such as developing a wind-down time every night before bed. Or you could stop having a second latte. Once you've got your new habits down and are able to do them consistently, chip away at another new habit.

You can keep implementing your new habits this way until you've gone through the full list in your goal-setting matrix. Then it's time to re-evaluate your goals. Are you where you want to be? Is there anything else that you could do to be healthier? What changes can you make today that will help you reach those goals? You've got an entire lifetime to keep working at developing new lifestyle strategies.

It's also important not to get too goal-driven. It is a delicate balance between having goals to stay motivated and using them to rule your life. I still want you to have flexibility so that you don't feel like you must adhere to a specific set of rules. Come up with habits that are realistic for you to stick to. And remember to have fun along the way.

Identify How

What do you need to do to achieve your lifestyle goals? You might have the best of intentions but no idea where you need to start to accomplish your goals. Start by brainstorming ideas that *might* work. There are no bad ideas here! Maybe you need to do some more reading on a specific topic, research a personal trainer in your area, or get counseling to deal with an unresolved emotional issue. What skills do you need to develop? How can you get there?

Making lifestyle changes can be difficult and challenging. Recruit a support team to help you out. Surround yourself with a team of experts that you rely on for accurate information. They may include your doctor, a psychologist, a dietician, a physiotherapist, a dentist, a personal trainer, a coach, or many others. Find a role model or mentor who can help keep you on track. Make sure that those you turn to rely on achieving results without quick-fix solutions.

Create Success

By this point, you should have pretty much everything that you need to create a lifestyle filled with health, energy, and vitality. To help keep you on track, you can journal your progress and keep track of the changes that you've successfully implemented. Rather than getting caught up in your struggles (because they will happen), focus on what you've done, sort of like a gratitude journal. Each day, write down one thing that you did in line with the goal of creating a healthier life. When you are having a bad day, you'll be able to look at all the good you've done as motivation to get back on track.

Another thing that can keep you on track is a lifestyle vision board. This collage is a great way to help you visualize where you would like to be. Go through your favorite magazines or pull images off the internet that are in line with your greater goals. Include other key aspects to your success on this board such as family support, healthy foods, fitness goals, dreams, or activities that you've always wanted to try. Fill your board with a variety of pictures and words that motivate you to stay on track. Hang your lifestyle vision board somewhere you see it often, and look at it for inspiration.

The last activity I want to leave you with is to read your goals daily. By keeping your goals at the front of your mind, you'll be more likely to accomplish them. Post your goals in a place where you'll see every day and read them out loud to yourself. Keep them updated as you successfully accomplish them. I've accomplished so much more by having a goal board, and I encourage you to do the same. To download a PDF of my free Goal Setting Guide that you can use to set your daily health goals, go to:

www.yourlifestylestrategy.com/bookbonus

As you embark on your own health journey, know that you already come equipped with everything you need to get started. You are **not** broken. You do **not** need to be fixed. It's time to stop making excuses and start taking charge of your health. It won't always be perfect, but keep trying anyway.

Know that I'm right there alongside you on your journey, cheering you on!

In health!

Shawna

Appendix

Date		Monday	Tuesday	Wednesday	Thursday	Friday	Saturday	Sunday
A	I napped for (xxx) minutes yesterday:							
B	Sleep aids I took last night:							
C	List any caffeine, nicotine, alcohol, drugs consumed today:							
D	I went to bed at (xxx) time:							
E	I turned off the light intending to sleep after (xxx) minutes:							
F	From the time I started trying to sleep, it took (xxx) minutes to fall asleep:							
G	My planned wake-up time this morning: (write none if you didn't have one)							
H	My actual final wake-up time this morning: (no more sleep after this)							
I	Time I got out of bed:							
J	"Number of times I woke up in the night: (write "0" if you did not wake up)"							
K	How long, all together, was I awake in the middle of the night? (minutes)							
L	Total Minutes in Bed Time between D + I							
M	Total minutes awake (Row E + F + K)							
N	How many minutes sleep did I get last night? (Row L – Row M) (Goal: 420–540)							
O	Sleep Efficiency [(Row L-M)/L]x 100= %							
P	Quality of sleep: 1=very poor, 10=excellent							
	Notes:							

Quick-Start Meal Guide

For those of you who need a little bit more support to get started, here are a few incredibly simple ideas for each meal to start you out. You don't need to be a master in the kitchen to make these recipes. For more recipes and ideas on what to eat, please refer to the recipes section of my website at www.yourlifestylestrategy.com. If you have healthy recipes that you'd like me to share with others, please send them to me through my website.

Breakfast

Easy Omelet

Ingredients: • 4–5 cups of seasonal vegetables
• 1 dozen eggs

Directions: • Sauté vegetables until the water starts to get released. Pour off liquids and then lay vegetables evenly in a lasagna pan lined with tinfoil or parchment paper
• Scramble a dozen eggs and pour them on top of the vegetables
• Bake for 30 minutes at 350°F or until eggs are firm

Salmon Avocado Salad

Ingredients: • Leftover salmon or canned salmon

• ½ English cucumber

• 1 avocado

• Juice from ½ lemon

Directions: • Drain water from can of salmon or flake leftover salmon and place in a small mixing bowl

• Dice ½ of an English cucumber and add to bowl

• Cut avocado in half and mash up the half without the pit, adding to bowl. Cover the other half for later use

• Stir together lemon juice, cucumber, mashed avocado and salmon

• Enjoy!

Breakfast Hash

Ingredients: • 1 lb potato or sweet potato

• 1 lb lean ground meat (chicken, turkey or pork)

• 3 cups mixed veggies (e.g., mushrooms, onions, peppers)

• 1 tbsp each of spices (cinnamon and mild curry)

Directions: • Brown ground meat

• While meat is browning, grate potato or sweet potato and rough chop mixed veggies

• Drain most of the fat from meat, leaving a tablespoon to cook your other ingredients

• Add potato, veggies, and spices to meat and sauté until cooked

Lunch

Kitchen Sink Salad

Ingredients: • Leftover protein
• Mixed salad greens
• ½ lemon
• Olive Oil

Directions: • Fill a large bowl with mixed salad greens
• Top with leftover protein from dinner
• Squeeze on the juice from ½ a lemon and add a drizzle of olive oil

Leftovers!

Seriously—this is the easiest way to eat lunch. When you are making dinner, prepare extra portions so that you have enough food to eat the next day. Eat it warm. Eat it cold. Doesn't really matter. Eating leftovers will save you a ton of time in food prep.

Dinner

Pork Loin and Veggies

Ingredients: • Pork loin
• Baby potatoes
• 1 bundle of asparagus
• 1 tsp each of thyme, pepper, garlic powder
• Salt and pepper to taste
• 1 tbsp coconut oil
• 1 cup chicken broth (homemade is best if you have it)

Directions: • Season pork loin with spices
• Turn on slow cooker with pork loin and chicken broth on low for 6–8 hours (while you are busy with other things!)
• When you are home from work, toss baby potatoes with coconut oil, salt, and pepper

- Bake in the oven at 350°F until potatoes are soft
- Lightly grill asparagus on the barbecue when the potatoes are almost done

Seasonal White Fish

Ingredients:
- ½ of white fish
- 4 cups mixed seasonal vegetables
- Fresh herbs, Italian seasoning, and pepper to taste
- ½ lemon
- 1 tsp butter

Directions:
- Place fish skin-side down on tinfoil, season with herbs and lemon juice. Seal package.
- In another tinfoil package, season chopped veggies with Italian seasoning, pepper, and butter
- Bake or barbecue both foil packages for the same amount of time
- This meal has a super easy clean-up!

Slow-Cooked Roast Beef

Ingredients:
- Beef roast or brisket
- 1 cup wild rice
- 4 cups fresh green beans
- 1 tsp each of smoked alder salt, pepper, garlic powder
- 1 cup beef broth (homemade is best if you have it)

Directions:
- Toss your beef roast in your mixed spices. Place into a roasting pan, add beef broth, and cover with tinfoil.
- Bake in the oven at 275°F until beef hits desired temperature
- Once meat is 10 degrees away from desired temperature, put wild rice into the rice cooker and put a tray of green beans in the top basket to steam
- Remove meat from oven when at desired temperature and set aside to rest until rice cooker is finished
- Slice meat thin and serve with rice and green beans

References

Sleep

Bonnet, M. H., & Arand, D. L. (2015). Overview of insomnia. Retrieved October 25, 2015, from http://www.uptodate.com/contents/overview-of-insomnia?source=search_result&search=sleep&selectedTitle=10~150

Bonnet, M. H., & Arand, D. L. (2015). Treatment of insomnia. Retrieved October 25, 2015, from http://www.uptodate.com/contents/treatment-of-insomnia?source=search_result&search=sleep&selectedTitle=27~150

Bonnet, M. H., & Arand, D. L. (2015). Patient information: insomnia treatments beyond the basics. Retrieved October 25, 2015, from http://www.uptodate.com/contents/insomnia-treatments-beyond-the-basics?source=search_result&search=sleep+hygeine&selectedTitle=5~150

Bonnie, R. J., & George, C. F. (2013). Liabilities of sleep deprivation and sleep disorders. Retrieved October 25, 2015, from http://www.uptodate.com/contents/liabilities-of-sleep-deprivation-and-sleep-disorders?source=search_result&search=sleep&selectedTitle=48~150

Bonnie, R. J., & George, C. F. (2015). Performance and safety risks of sleep deprivation and sleep disorders. Retrieved October 25, 2015, from http://www.uptodate.com/contents/performance-and-safety-risks-of-sleep-deprivation-and-sleep-disorders?source=search_result&search=sleep&selectedTitle=22~150

Chervin, R. D. (2015). Approach to the patient with excessive daytime sleepiness. Retrieved October 25, 2015, from http://www.uptodate.com/contents/approach-to-the-patient-with-excessive-daytime-sleepiness?source=search_result&search=sleep&selectedTitle=26~150

Cirelli, C. (2015). Sleep insufficiency: definition, consequences, and management. Retrieved October 25, 2015, from http://www.uptodate.com/contents/sleep-insufficiency-definition-consequences-and-management?source=search_result&search=sleep&selectedTitle=4~150

Conley, S., & Redeker, N. S. (2015). Cognitive behavioral therapy for insomnia in the context of cardiovascular conditions. *Current Sleep Medicine Reports, 1*, 157–165. http://doi.org/10.1007/s40675-015-0019-7

Drake, C. L., & Cheng, P. (2015). Sleep-wake disturbances in shift workers. Retrieved October 25, 2015, from http://www.uptodate.com/contents/sleep-wake-disturbances-in-shift-workers?source=search_result&search=sleep&selectedTitle=3~150

Driver, H. S. (2012). Sleepless women: insomnia from the female perspective. *Insomnia Rounds, 1*(6).

Ellenbogen, J. M. (2005). Cognitive benefits of sleep and their loss due to sleep deprivation. *Neurology, 64*, E25-7.

Foldvary-Schaefer, N. (2015). Disorders of arousal from non-rapid eye movement sleep in adults. Retrieved October 25, 2015, from http://www.uptodate.com/contents/disorders-of-arousal-from-non-rapid-eye-movement-sleep-in-adults?source=search_result&search=sleep&selectedTitle=6~150

Freedman, N. (2015). Quantifying sleepiness. Retrieved October 25, 2015, from http://www.uptodate.com/contents/quantifying-sleepiness?source=search_result&search=sleep&selectedTitle=47~150

Hanlon, E. C., Tasali, E., Leproult, R., Stuhr, K. L., Doncheck, E., De Wit, H., ... Cauter, E. V. (2016). Sleep duration/sleep quality: sleep restriction enhances the daily rhythm of circulating levels of endocannabinoid 2-arachidonoylglycerol. *Sleep, 39*(3). http://doi.org/10.5665/sleep.5546

Irwin, M. R., Olmstead, R., & Motivala, S. J. (2008). Thai chi chih and sleep quality in the elderly: improving sleep quality in older adults with moderate sleep complaints: a randomized control trial of tai chi chih. *Sleep, 31*(7), 1001–1008.

Jacobs, G. D. (1998). Say good night to insomnia: a drug-free program developed at Harvard medical school. New York: Holt Paperbacks.

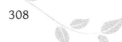

Judd, B. G., & Sateia, M. J. (2015). Classification of sleep disorders. Retrieved October 25, 2015, from http://www.uptodate.com/contents/classification-of-sleep-disorders?source=search_result&search=sleep&selectedTitle=9~150

Kirsch, D. (2015). Stages and architecture of normal sleep. Retrieved October 25, 2015, from http://www.uptodate.com/contents/stages-and-architecture-of-normal-sleep?source=search_result&search=sleep&selectedTitle=2~150

Kryger, M. H. (2004). *Can't sleep, can't stay awake* (First). Toronto: Harper Collins Publishers Ltd.

Liu, R., Liu, X., Zee, P. C., Hou, L., Zheng, Z., Wei, Y., ... Zheng, H. L. (2014). Association between sleep quality and c-reactive protein: results from national health and nutrition examination survey, 2005-2008. *PLoS ONE*, 9(3). http://doi.org/10.1371/journal.pone.0092607

Meoli, A. L., Rosen, C., Kristo, D., Kohrman, M., Gooneratne, N., Aguillard, R. N., ... Mahowald, M. (2005). Oral nonprescription treatment for insomnia: an evaluation of products with limited evidence. *Journal of Clinical Sleep Medicine*, 1(2), 173–187.

National Sleep Foundation. (2015). Shift work disorder: non-medical treatments for shift work disorder. Retrieved November 16, 2015, from https://sleepfoundation.org/shift-work/content/non-medical-treatments-shift-work-disorder

National Sleep Foundation. (2015). Electronics in the bedroom: why it's necessary to turn off before you tuck in. Retrieved November 16, 2015, from https://sleepfoundation.org/ask-the-expert/electronics-the-bedroom

Robertson, E. M., Pascual-Leone, A., & Press, D. Z. (2004). Awareness modifies the skill-learning benefits of sleep. *Current Biology*, 14, 208–212. http://doi.org/10.1016/j.cub.2004.01.027

Roehrs, T., & Roth, T. (2015). The effects of medications on sleep quality and sleep architecture. Retrieved October 25, 2015, from http://www.uptodate.com/contents/the-effects-of-medications-on-sleep-quality-and-sleep-architecture?source=search_result&search=sleep&selectedTitle=12~150

Roizenblatt, M., Rosa Neto, N. S., Tufik, S., & Roizenblatt, S. (2012). Pain-related diseases and sleep disorders. *Brazilian Journal of Medical and Biological Research*, 45(9), 792–798. http://doi.org/10.1590/S0100-879X2012007500110

Schutte-Rodin, S., Broch, L., Buysse, D., Dorsey, C., & Sateia, M. (2008). Clinical guideline for the evaluation and management of chronic insomnia in adults. *Journal of Clinical Sleep Medicine, 4*(5).

Silva-Costa, A., Griep, R. H., & Rotenberg, L. (2015). Disentangling the effects of insomnia and night work on cardiovascular diseases: a study in nursing professionals. *Brazilian Journal of Medical and Biological Research, 48*(2), 120–127. http://doi.org/10.1590/1414-431X20143965

Strohl, K. P. (2015). Overview of obstructive sleep apnea in adults. Retrieved October 25, 2015, from http://www.uptodate.com/contents/overview-of-obstructive-sleep-apnea-in-adults?source=search_result&search=sleep&selectedTitle=13~150

Toward Optimized Practice. (2015). *Adult insomnia: assessment to management.* Edmonton. Retrieved from http://www.topalbertadoctors.org/download/1920/Adult Insomnia CPG.pdf?_20170125205043

Vaughn, B. V. (2015). Approach to abnormal movements and behaviors during sleep. Retrieved October 30, 2015, from http://www.uptodate.com/contents/approach-to-abnormal-movements-and-behaviors-during-sleep?source=search_result&search=sleep&selectedTitle=11~150

Smith, T. J. (2009). Magnesium supplements for menopausal hot flashes. *American Society of Clinical Oncology, 27*(7), 1151–1152. http://doi.org/10.1200/JCO.2009.21.3629

The doctors and editors at UptoDate. (2015). Patient information: insomnia: the basics. Retrieved October 25, 2015, from http://www.uptodate.com/contents/insomnia-the-basics?source=search_result&search=sleep+hygiene&selectedTitle=2~62

Vyazovskiy, V. V. (2015). Sleep, recovery, and metaregulation: explaining the benefits of sleep. *Nature and Science of Sleep, 7*, 171–184. http://doi.org/10.2147/NSS.S54036

Watson, N. F., Badr, M. S., Belenky, G., Bliwise, D. L., Buxton, O. M., Buysse, D., ... Heald, J. L. (2015). Recommended amount of sleep for a healthy adult: a joint consensus statement of the american academy of sleep medicine and sleep research society. *Journal of Clinical Sleep Medicine, 11*(6), 591–591. http://doi.org/10.5664/jcsm.4758

Nutrition

Alberta Health Services. (2013). *Nutrition guideline: adult weight management.* Retrieved from http://www.albertahealthservices.ca/assets/Infofor/hp/if-hp-ed-cdm-ns-5-6-1-adult-weight-management.pdf

Alexander, D. D., Cushing, C. A., & Alexander, D. D. (2010). Red meat and colorectal cancer: a critical summary of prospective epidemiologic studies. *International Association for the Study of Obesity, 12*(5), e472–e493. http://doi.org/10.1111/j.1467-789X.2010.00785.x

Atkins, J. L., Whincup, P. H., Morris, R. W., Lennon, L. T., Papacosta, O., & Goya Wannamethee, S. (2014). High diet quality is associated with a lower risk of cardiovascular disease and all-cause mortality in older men. *Journal of Nutrition, 144,* 673–680. http://doi.org/10.3945/jn.113.186486

Ball, R. O. (2015). Protein requirements: time to re-evaluate canadian recommendations. Retrieved December 15, 2015, from https://www.dairynutrition.ca/scientific-evidence/experts-summaries/protein-requirements-time-to-re-evaluate-canadian-recommendations

Bolland, M., Tai, V., Leung, W., Grey, A., Reid, I. R., & Bolland, M. J. (2015). Stratification of risk for hospital admissions for injury related to fall: cohort study. *BMJ, 351.* http://doi.org/10.1136/bmj.h4183

Burke, L. M., Cox, G. R., Cummings, N. K., & Desbrow, B. (2001). Guidelines for daily carbohydrate intake: do athletes achieve them ? *Sports Medicine, 31*(4), 267–299. http://doi.org/10.2165/00007256-200131040-00003

Colditz, G. A. (2015). Healthy diet in adults. Retrieved October 8, 2015, from http://www.uptodate.com/contents/healthy-diet-in-adults?source=search_result&search=healthy+diets+in+adults&selectedTitle=1~83

Cordain, L., Eaton, S. B., Sebastian, A., Mann, N., Lindeberg, S., Watkins, B. A., ... Brand-Miller, J. (2005). Origins and evolution of the western diet: health implications for the 21st century. *The American Journal of Clinical Nutrition, 81,* 341–54.

Dairy Nutrition. (2015). Sustainable diets 101. Retrieved December 15, 2015, from https://www.dairynutrition.ca/sustainable-diets-101

Delahanty, L. M., & McCulloch, D. K. (2015). Nutritional considerations in type 2 diabetes mellitus. Retrieved October 8, 1015, from http://www.uptodate.com/contents/nutritional-considerations-in-type-2-diabetes-mellitus?source=search_result&search=nutritional+considerations+in+type+2&selectedTitle=1~150

DeLegge, M. H. (2015). Nutrition and dietary interventions in adults with inflammatory bowel disease. Retrieved October 8, 2015, from http://www.uptodate.com/contents/nutrition-and-dietary-interventions-in-adults-with-inflammatory-bowel-disease?source=search_result&search=nutrition+and+dietary+interventions&selectedTitle=1~150

Demory-Luce, D., & Motil, K. J. (2015). Fast food for children and adolescents. Retrieved October 8, 2015, from http://www.uptodate.com/contents/fast-food-for-children-and-adolescents?source=search_result&search=food+availability&selectedTitle=4~150

Drewnowski, A. (2015). Building healthier diets: the nutrient-rich foods index. Retrieved December 5, 2015, from https://www.dairynutrition.ca/scientific-evidence/experts-summaries/building-healthier-diets-the-nutrient-rich-foods-index

Fairfield, K. M. (2015). Vitamin supplementation in disease prevention. Retrieved October 8, 2015, from http://www.uptodate.com/contents/vitamin-supplementation-in-disease-prevention?source=search_result&search=vitamin+supplementation&selectedTitle=1~150

Forsythe, C. E., Phinney, S. D., Feinman, R. D., Volk, B. M., Freidenreich, D., Quann, E., ... Volek, J. S. (2010). Limited effect of dietary saturated fat on plasma saturated fat in the context of a low carbohydrate diet. *Lipids*, 45(10), 947–62. http://doi.org/DOI 10.1007/s11745-010-3467-3

Gillman, M. W. (2014). Dietary fat. Retrieved October 8, 2015, from http://www.uptodate.com/contents/dietary-fat?source=search_result&search=dietary+fat&selectedTitle=1~101

Government of Alberta. (2016). *Alberta nutrition guidelines for adults*. Retrieved from http://www.health.alberta.ca/documents/Nutrition-Guidelines-AB-Adults.pdf

Groetch, M. (2015). Management of food allergy: nutritional issues. Retrieved October 8, 2015, from http://www.uptodate.com/contents/management-of-food-allergy-nutritional-issues?source=search_result&search=management+of+food+allergies&selectedTitle=4~150

Haas, E. M., & Levin, B. (2006). Staying healthy with nutrition: the complete guide to diet and nutritional medicine: 21st century edition. Berkeley: Celestial Arts.

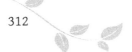

Haring, B., Gronroos, N., Nettleton, J., Wyler von Ballmoos, M. C., Selvin, E., & Alonso, A. (2014). Dietary protein intake and coronary heart disease in a large community based cohor: results from the atherosclerosis risk in communities (ARIC) study. *PLOS ONE, 9*(10). Retrieved from https://www.ncbi.nlm.nih.gov/pubmed/25303709

Health Canada. (2007). Eating well with canada's food guide. Her Majesty the Queen in Right of Canada, represented by the Minister of Health Canada. Retrieved from http://www.hc-sc.gc.ca/fn-an/food-guide-aliment/index-eng.php

Health Canada. (2008). *Nutrient value of some common foods.* Ottawa: Minister of Health.

Hite, A. H., Goldstein Berkowitz, V., & Berkowitz, K. (2011). Low-carbohydrate diet review: shifting the paradigm. *Nutrition in Clinical Practice, 26*(3), 300–308. http://doi.org/10.1177/0884533611405791

Ho, V. W., Leung, K., Hsu, A., Luk, B., Lai, J., Shen, S. Y., ... Krystal, G. (2001). A low carbohydrate, high protein diet slows tumor growth and prevents cancer initiation. *American Association for Cancer Research, 71*(13), 4480–4493. http://doi.org/10.1158/0008-5472.CAN-10-3973

Hoch, T., Kreitz, S., Gaffling, S., Pischetsrieder, M., & Hess, A. (2015). Fat/carbohydrate ratio but not energy density determines snack food intake and activates brain reward areas. *Nature Publishing Group.* http://doi.org/10.1038/srep10041

Hu, F. B. (2010). Are refined carbohydrates worse than saturated fat? *American Clinical Journal of Nutrition, 91*(6), 1541–2. http://doi.org/10.3945/ajcn.2010.29622

Institute of Medicine of the National Academies. (2005). *Dietary reference intakes for energy, carbohydrate. fiber, fat, fatty acids, cholesterol, protein, and amino acids.* Washington: National Academies Press. Retrieved from http://www.nap.edu/search/?term=Dietary+Reference+Intakes%3A+Macronutrients

Kaplan, N. M., & Forman, J. P. (2015). Diet in the treatment and prevention of hypertension. Retrieved October 8, 2015, from http://www.uptodate.com/contents/diet-in-the-treatment-and-prevention-of-hypertension?source=search_result&search=diet+in+treatment+and+prevention+of+hypertension&selectedTitle=1~150

Kossoff, E. H. W. (2015). The ketogenic diet. Retrieved October 8, 2015, from http://www.uptodate.com/contents/the-ketogenic-diet?source=search_result&search=the+ketogenic+diet&selectedTitle=1~36

Layman, D. K., Boileau, R. A., Erickson, D. J., Painter, J. E., Shiue, H., Sather, C., & Christou, D. D. (2003). Human nutrition and metabolism: a reduced ratio of dietary carbohydrate to protein improves body composition and blood lipid profiles during weight loss in adult women. *Journal of Nutrition, 133*, 411–417.

Layman, D. K., Evans, E., Baum, J. I., Seyler, J., Erickson, D. J., & Boileau, R. A. (2005). Human nutrition and metabolism: dietary protein and exercise have additive effects on body composition during weight loss in adult women. *Journal of Nutrition, 135*, 1903–1910.

Liu, S., & Willett, W. C. (2014). Dietary carbohydrates. Retrieved October 8, 2015, from http://www.uptodate.com/contents/dietary-carbohydrates?source=search_result&search=dietary+carbohydrates&selectedTitle=1~70

Maki, K. C., Van Elswyk, M. E., Alexander, D. D., Rains, T. M., Sohn, E. L., & McNeill, S. (2012). A meta-analysis of randomized controlled trials that compare the lipid effects of beef versus poultry and/or fish consumption. *Journal of Clinical Lipidology, 6*(4), 352–361. http://doi.org/10.1016/j.jacl.2012.01.001

Manninen, A. H. (2004). Metabolic effects of the very-low-carbohydrate diets: misunderstood "villains" of human metabolism. *Journal of the International Society of Sports Nutrition. Journal of the International Society of Sports Nutrition, 1*(12), 7–117.

Martens, E. A., Tan, S. Y., Dunlop, M. V., Mattes, R. D., & Westerterp-Plantenga, M. S. (2014). Protein leverage effects of beef protein on energy intake in humans. *The American Journal of Clinical Nutrition, 99*, 1397–406. http://doi.org/10.3945/ajcn.113.078774

Mattson, M. P., Allison, D. B., Fontana, L., Harvie, M., Longo, V. D., Malaisse, W. J., ... Panda, S. (2014). Meal frequency and timing in health and disease. *Proceedings of the National Academy of Sciences of the United States of America, 111*(47), 11647–11653. http://doi.org/10.1073/pnas.1413965111

Melnik, B. C., John, S. M., & Schmitz, G. (2011). Over-stimulation of insulin/igf-1 signaling by western diet may promote diseases of civilization: lessons learnt from laron syndrome. *Nutrition and Metabolism, 41*(8). Retrieved from http://www.nutritionandmetabolism.com/content/8/1/41

Mente, A., de Koning, L., Shannon, H. S., & Anand, S. S. (2009). A systematic review of the evidence supporting a causal link between dietary factors and coronary heart disease. *Archives of Internal Medicine, 169*(7), 659–669. http://doi.org/10.1001/archinternmed.2009.38

Micha, R., Wallace, S. K., & Mozaffarian, D. (2010). Epidemiology and prevention red and processed meat consumption and risk of incident coronary heart disease, stroke, and diabetes mellitus: a systematic review and meta-analysis. *American Heart Association, 121*, 2271–2283. http://doi.org/10.1161/CIRCULATIONAHA.109.924977

Niagara Health System. (2012). An introduction to the low fodmap diet for irritable bowel syndrome.

Nutrition Working Group of the International Olympic Committee. (2012). *Nutrition for athletes: a practical guide to eating for health and performance.* Retrieved from http://www.olympic.org/documents/reports/en/en_report_833.pdf

Olendzski, B. (2013). Dietary and nutritional assessment in adults. Retrieved October 8, 2015, from http://www.uptodate.com/contents/dietary-and-nutritional-assessment-in-adults?source=search_result&search=dietary+and+nutritional+assessment+in+adults&selectedTitle=1~150

Panandiker, D. H. P., Satyanarayana, K., Ramana, Y. V., Sinha, R., Grandjean, A. C., Harris, S., & Sharma, R. (2007). *Nutrition and hydration guidelines for excellence in sports performance.* Bangalor. Retrieved from http://www.ilsi-india.org/PDF/Conf. recommendations/Nutrition/Nutrition & Hyd. Guidelines for Athletes Final report.pdf

Phillips, S. M., Fulgoni III, V. L., Heaney, R. P., Nicklas, T. A., Slavin, J. L., & Weaver, C. M. (2015). Commonly consumed protein foods contribute to nutrient intake, diet quality, and nutrient adequacy. *American Journal of Clinical Nutrition, 101*, 1317S–1319S. http://doi.org/10.3945/ajcn.114.084079

Popkin, B. M., D'anci, K. E., & Rosenberg, I. H. (2010). Water, hydration and health. *Nutrition Review, 68*(8), 30. http://doi.org/10.1111/j.1753-4887.2010.00304.x

Ritchie, C., & Yukawa, M. (2015). Geriatric nutrition: nutritional issues in older adults. Retrieved January 26, 2016, from http://www.uptodate.com/contents/geriatric-nutrition-nutritional-issues-in-older-adults?source=search_result&search=marijuana&selectedTitle=22~150

Rodriguez, N. R. (2015). Introduction to protein summit 2.0: continued exploration of the impact of high-quality protein on optimal health. *Journal of Clinical Nutrition, 101,* 1317s–19s. http://doi.org/10.3945/ajcn.114.083980

Rohrmann, S., Overvad, K., Bas Bueno-De-Mesquita, H., Jakobsen, M. U., Egeberg, R., Tjønneland, A., ... Linseisen, J. (2013). Meat consumption and mortality -results from the european prospective investigation into cancer and nutrition. *BMC Medicine, 63*(11). Retrieved from http://www.biomedcentral.com/1741-7015/11/63

Rosenberg, I. H. (1994). Human nutrient requirements nutrient requirements for optimal health: what does that mean? *Journal of Nutrition, 124,* 1777s–1779s.

Roussell, M. A., Hill, A. M., Gaugler, T. L., West, S. G., Vanden Heuvel, J. P., Alaupovic, P., ... Kris-Etherton, P. M. (2012). Beef in an optimal lean diet study: effects on lipids, lipoproteins, and apolipoproteins. *American Journal of Clinical Nutrition, 95,* 9–16. http://doi.org/10.3945/ajcn.111.016261

Sawka, M. N., Burke, L. M., Eichner, E. R., Maughan, R. J., Montain, S. J., & Stachenfield, N. S. (2007). Exercise and fluid replacement. *American College of Sports Medicine, 32*(2), 377–390. http://doi.org/10.1249/mss.0b013e31802ca597

Sluijs, I., Van Der Schouw, Y. T., Van Der A, D. L., Spijkerman, A. M., Hu, F. B., Grobbee, D. E., & Beulens, J. W. (2010). Carbohydrate quantity and quality and risk of type 2 diabetes in the European Prospective Investigation into Cancer and Nutrition–Netherlands (EPIC-NL) study 1–3. *The American Journal of Clinical Nutrition, 92,* 905–911. http://doi.org/10.3945/ajcn.2010.29620

Spreadbury, I. (2012). Diabetes, metabolic syndrome and obesity: targets and therapy. *Diabetes, Metabolic Syndrome and Obesity: Targets and Therapy, 5,* 175–189. http://doi.org/10.2147/DMSO.S33473

Sterns, R. H. (2014). Maintenance and replacement fluid therapy in adults. Retrieved October 8, 2015, from http://www.uptodate.com/contents/maintenance-and-replacement-fluid-therapy-in-adults?source=search_result&search=maintainance+and+replacement+fluid+therapy&selectedTitle=1~150

Tangney, C. C., & Rosenson, R. S. (2015). Lipid lowering with diet or dietary supplements. Retrieved October 8, 2015, from http://www.uptodate.com/contents/lipid-lowering-with-diet-or-dietary-supplements?source=search_result&search=lipid+lowering+diet&selectedTitle=1~150

Toward Optimized Practice Working Group for Vitamin D. (2012). *Guideline for vitamin d testing and supplementation in adults*. Edmonton. Retrieved from http://www.topalbertadoctors.org/cpgs/?sid=18&cpg_cats=91

Volek, J. S., Quann, E. E., & Forsythe, C. E. (2010). Low carbohydrate diets promote a more favorable body composition than low-fat diets. *National Strength and Conditioning Association, 32*(1), 42–47.

Wurtman, R. J., Wurtman, J. J., Regan, M. M., Mcdermott, J. M., Tsay, R. H., & Breu, J. J. (2003). Effects of normal meals rich in carbohydrates or proteins on plasma tryptophan and tyrosine ratios 1–3. *American Journal of Clinical Nutrition, 77*, 128–32.

Exercise

American Academy of Orthopaedic Surgeons. (2013). *Healthy bones at every age*. Retrieved from www.orthoinfo.org

Burton, E., Cavalheri, V., Adams, R., Oakley Browne, C., Bovery-Spencer, P., Fenton, A. M., ... Hill, K. D. (2015). Effectiveness of exercise programs to reduce falls in older people with dementia living in the community: a systematic review and meta-analysis. *Dove Press Journal, 10*, 421–434. http://doi.org/10.2147/CIA.S71691

Canadian Nurses Association. (2011). Promoting physical activity: brief to the house of commons standing committee on health. Ottawa.

Canadian Society for Exercise Physiology. (2012). Canadian physical activity guidelines and sedentary behaviour guidelines: your plan to get active every day. Retrieved from www.csep.ca/guidelines

Chen, H., Zhou, X., Fujita, H., Onozuka, M., & Kubo, K. (2013). Age-related changes in trabecular and cortical bone microstructure. *International Journal of Endocrinology, 2013*(213234), 1–9. http://doi.org/10.1155/2013/213234

Crohn's & Colitis Foundation of America. (2012). Bone loss. Retrieved from http://www.ccfa.org/resources/bone-loss.html?referrer=https://www.google.ca/

Daly, R. M., Rosengren, B. E., Alwis, G., Ahlborg, H. G., Sernbo, I., & Karlsson, M. K. (2013). Gender specific age-related changes in bone density, muscle strength and functional performance in the elderly: a-10 year prospective population-based study. *BMC Geriatrics, 71*(13), 2–9. Retrieved from http://www.biomedcentral.com/1471-2318/13/71

Douglas, P. S. (2015). Exercise and fitness in the prevention of cardiovascular disease. Retrieved October 25, 2015, from http://www.uptodate.com/contents/exercise-and-fitness-in-the-prevention-of-cardiovascular-disease?source=search_result&search=exercise&selectedTitle=2~150

Fishbein, D. B., & Saper, R. B. (2015). Overview of yoga. *UpToDate.* Retrieved from http://www.uptodate.com/contents/overview-of-yoga?source=search_result&search=injury+prevention&selectedTitle=27~49

Gecht-Silver, M. R., & Duncombe, A. M. (2015). Overview of joint protection. Retrieved October 25, 2015, from http://www.uptodate.com/contents/overview-of-joint-protection?source=search_result&search=exercise&selectedTitle=40~150

Howard, T. M. (2015). Overtraining syndrome in athletes. Retrieved October 25, 2015, from http://www.uptodate.com/contents/overtraining-syndrome-in-athletes?source=search_result&search=cardiovascular+training&selectedTitle=1~150

Keating, S. E., George, J., & Johnson, N. A. (2015). The benefits of exercise for patients with non-alcoholic fatty liver disease. *Expert Review of Gastroenterology & Hepatology, 9*(10), 1247–1250. http://doi.org/10.1586/17474124.2015.1075392

Morey, M. C. (2015). Physical activity and exercise in older adults. Retrieved October 30, 2015, from http://www.uptodate.com/contents/physical-activity-and-exercise-in-older-adults?source=search_result&search=exercise&selectedTitle=4~150

National Institutes of Health. (2015). Osteoporosis: peak bone mass in women. NIH Osteoporosis and Related Bone Diseases National Resource Centre. Bethesda. Retrieved from www.bones.nih.gov

O'Flaherty, E. J. (2000). Modeling normal aging bone loss, with consideration of bone loss in osteoporosis. *Toxicology Sciences,* (55), 171–188.

Peterson, D. M. (2015). The benefits and risks of exercise. Retrieved October 30, 2015, from http://www.uptodate.com/contents/the-benefits-and-risks-of-exercise?source=search_result&search=exercise&selectedTitle=1~150

Peterson, D. M. (2015). Patient information—beyond the basics. Retrieved October 30, 2015, from http://www.uptodate.com/contents/exercise-beyond-the-basics?source=see_link

Peterson, D. M. (2015). Patient information: exercise (the basics). Retrieved October 30, 2015, from http://www.uptodate.com/contents/exercise-the-basics?source=search_result&search=exercise&selectedTitle=3~150

Powers, S. K., & Dodd, S. L. (1996). *Total fitness exercise, nutrition and wellness* (First). Needham Heights: Allyn and Bacon.

Skinner, J. S. (2005). Exercise testing and exercise prescription for special cases: theoretical basis and clinical application (Second). Philadelphia: Lippincott Williams & Wilkins.

Systrom, D. M., & Lewis, G. D. (2015). Exercise physiology. Retrieved October 25, 2015, from http://www.uptodate.com/contents/exercise-physiology?source=search_result&search=exercise&selectedTitle=7~150

Mental Health

Ameringen, M. V. (2015). Comorbid anxiety and depression: epidemiology, clinical manifestations, and diagnosis. Retrieved October 25, 2015, from http://www.uptodate.com/contents/comorbid-anxiety-and-depression-epidemiology-clinical-manifestations-and-diagnosis?source=search_result&search=depression&selectedTitle=16~150

Burns, D. D. (2000). *Feeling good the new mood therapy.* New York: HarperCollins Publishers Inc.

Bystritsky, A. (2015). Complementary and alternative treatments for anxiety symptoms and disorders: physical, cognitive, and spiritual interventions. Retrieved October 25, 2015, from http://www.uptodate.com/contents/complementary-and-alternative-treatments-for-anxiety-symptoms-and-disorders-physical-cognitive-and-spiritual-interventions?source=search_result&search=anxiety&selectedTitle=2~150

Carlson, N. R., Buskist, W., Enzle, M. E., & Heth, C. D. (2000). *Psychology: the science of behaviour* (Canadian). Scarborough: Allyth and Bacon Canada.

Greenberg, J. S. (1999). *Comprehensive stress management.* (E. E. Bartell & S. R. Oberbroeckling, Eds.) (Sixth). Boston: WCB McGraw Hill.

Levenson, J. L. (2015). Psychological factors affecting other medical conditions: clinical features, assessment, and diagnosis. Retrieved October 25, 2015, from http://www.uptodate.com/contents/psychological-factors-affecting-other-medical-conditions-clinical-features-assessment-and-diagnosis?source=search_result&search=mental+stress&selectedTitle=1~150

Lu, P. H. (2014). The mental status examination in adults. Retrieved October 25, 2015, from http://www.uptodate.com/contents/the-mental-status-examination-in-adults?source=search_result&search=mental+health+assessment&selectedTitle=1~150

319

Mental Health Commission of Canada. (2010). *Making the Case for Investing in Mental Health in Canada.* Retrieved from http://www.mentalhealthcommission.ca/sites/default/files/2016-06/Investing_in_Mental_Health_FINAL_Version_ENG.pdf

National Centre for Complementary and Integrative Health. (2014). Meditation for health: what science says. Retrieved October 30, 2015, from https://nccih.nih.gov/health/providers/digest/meditation-science

Nauert, R. (2011). Taking breaks found to improve attention. Retrieved December 26, 2016, from http://psychcentral.com/news/2011/02/09/taking-breaks-found-to-improve-attention/23329.html

Project: Time Off. (2016). Americans waste record-setting 658 million vacation days. Retrieved December 26, 2016, from http://www.projecttimeoff.com/NEWS/PRESS-RELEASES/AMERICANS-WASTE-RECORD-SETTING-658-MILLION-VACATION-DAYS

Sapolsky, R. M. (2004). Why zebras don't get ulcers: the acclaimed guide to stress, stress-related diseases and coping (Third). New York: Holt Paperbacks.

US Travel Association. (2014). Unused time off harms u.s. productivity, broader economy. Retrieved December 26, 2016, from https://www.ustravel.org/press/unused-time-harms-us-productivity-broader-economy

Williams, J., & Nieuwsma, J. (2015). Screening for depression. Retrieved October 25, 2015, from http://www.uptodate.com/contents/screening-for-depression?source=search_result&search=depression&selectedTitle=2~150

Digestion

Bollinger, T. (2016). Boost immunity with gut-immune-cancer connection. In *Where Health Starts and Your Healing Begins.* Axe Wellness, LLC. Retrieved from www.naturalgutcures.com

Bonis, P. A. L., Lamont, J. T., Rutgeerts, P., & Grover, S. (2015). Approach to the adult with chronic diarrhea in developed countries. Retrieved October 30, 2015, from http://www.uptodate.com/contents/approach-to-the-adult-with-chronic-diarrhea-in-developed-countries?source=search_result&search=chronic+diarrhea&selectedTitle=1~150

Cleveland Clinic. (2013). Keeping your digestive tract healthy. Retrieved October 30, 2015, from http://my.clevelandclinic.org/health/healthy_living/hic_Keeping_Your_Digestive_Tract_Healthy

Corliss, J., Elbaum, D. A., Long, G. J., & Villalba, C. (2015). Patient information: gas and bloating, the basics. Retrieved October 30, 2015, from http://www. uptodate.com/contents/gas-and-bloating-the-basics?source=search_result&search=flatulence&selectedTitle=3~150

Dethlefsena, L., & Relman, D. A. (2011). Incomplete recovery and individualized responses of the human distal gut microbiota to repeated antibiotic perturbation. *Proceedings of the National Academy of Sciences of the United States of America, 108*(1), 4554–4561. http://doi.org/10.1073/pnas.1000087107

Gill, H. S., & Guarner, F. (2004). Probiotics and human health: a clinical perspective. *Postgrad Medical Journal, 80*, 516–526. http://doi.org/10.1136/pgmj.2003.008664

Goldfinger, S. E., Lamont, J. T., & Grover, S. (2015). Patient information- gas and bloating, beyond the basics. Retrieved October 30, 2015, from http://www.uptodate.com/contents/gas-and-bloating-beyond-the-basics?source=search_result&search=flatulence&selectedTitle=2~150

Jardine, M. (2014). Seven foods to supercharge your gut bacteria. Retrieved October 30, 2015, from www.pcrm.org/media/online/sept2014/seven-foods-to-supercharge-your-gut-bacteria

Kresser, C. (2015). *Gut health.* Retrieved from www.chriskresser.com

Lacy, B. E., Gabbard, S. L., & Crowell, M. D. (2011). Pathophysiology, evaluation, and treatment of bloating: hope, hype, or hot air? *Gastroenterology & Hepatology, 7*(11), 729–39.

Mason, J. B., Lipman, T. O., & Grover, S. (2015). Mechanisms of nutrient absorption and malabsorption. Retrieved October 30, 2015, from http://www.uptodate.com/contents/mechanisms-of-nutrient-absorption-and-malabsorption?source=search_result&search=digestion&selectedTitle=1~142

Mason, J. B., Milovic, V., Lipman, T. O., & Grover, S. (2015). Clinical features and diagnosis of malabsorption. Retrieved October 30, 2015, from http://www.uptodate.com/contents/clinical-features-and-diagnosis-of-malabsorption?source=search_result&search=digestion&selectedTitle=3~142

Mason, J. B., Milovic, V., Lipman, T. O., & Grover, S. (2015). Overview of the treatment of malabsorption. Retrieved October 30, 2015, from http://www.uptodate.com/contents/overview-of-the-treatment-of-malabsorption?source=search_result&search=leaky+gut+syndrome&selectedTitle=7~109

Masterjohn, C. (2005). Cholesterol is necessary for digestion. Retrieved December 5, 2015, from http://www.cholesterol-and-health.com/search-cholesterol-and-health.html

Mayo Clinic Staff. (2015). Frequent bowel movements. Retrieved October 30, 2015, from http://www.mayoclinic.org/symptoms/frequent-bowel-movements/basics/definition/sym-20050720

Mercola, J. (2014). The secret behind bowel movements. Retrieved October 30, 2015, from http://articles.mercola.com/sites/articles/archive/2014/03/10/bowel-movements-segmentation.aspx

Mercola, J. (2015). Problems with digestion? Processed foods may be to blame. Retrieved October 30, 2015, from http://articles.mercola.com/sites/articles/archive/2011/01/06/what-you-need-to-understand-about-your-digestive-system-to-improve-your-health.aspx

Monastyrsky, K. (2015). How often should I move my bowels? Retrieved October 30, 2015, from https://www.gutsense.org/constipation/frequency.html

National Institute of Diabetes and Digestive and Kidney Diseases. (2013). Smoking and the digestive system. Retrieved October 30, 2015, from http://www.niddk.nih.gov/health-information/health-topics/digestive-diseases/smoking/Pages/facts.aspx

National Institute of Diabetes and Digestive and Kidney Diseases. (2014). Crohn's disease. Retrieved October 30, 2015, from http://www.niddk.nih.gov/health-information/health-topics/digestive-diseases/crohns-disease/Pages/facts.aspx

Pauley-Hunter, R. J., Vanderhoof, J. A., Lamont, J. T., & Motil, K. J. (2015). Pathophysiology of the short bowel syndrome. Retrieved October 30, 2015, from http://www.uptodate.com/contents/pathophysiology-of-the-short-bowel-syndrome?source=search_result&search=leaky+gut+syndrome&selectedTitle=2~109

Ruscio, M. (2015). Include cultured veggies on a leaky gut diet. Retrieved October 29, 2015, from http://drruscio.com/include-cultured-veggies-on-a-leaky-gut-diet/

Ruscio, M. (2015). Got allergies? Fix your gut. Retrieved October 29, 2015, from http://drruscio.com/got-allergies-fix-your-gut/

Ruscio, M. (2015). Ten things that can cause leaky gut. Retrieved October 29, 2015, from http://drruscio.com/ten-things-that-cause-leaky-gut/

Ruscio, M. (2015). What can cause constipation and what to do about it. Retrieved October 29, 2015, from http://drruscio.com/what-can-cause-constipation-and-what-to-do-about-it/

Sanderson, I., Klish, W. J., Motil, K. J., & Hoppin, A. G. (2015). Overview of the development of the gastrointestinal tract. Retrieved October 30, 2015, from http://www.uptodate.com/contents/overview-of-the-development-of-the-gastrointestinal-tract?source=search_result&search=digestion&selectedTitle=2~142

Schenker, S. (2015). Foods to improve digestion. Retrieved October 30, 2015, from http://www.ageuk.org.uk/health-wellbeing/healthy-eating-landing/foods-to-improve-digestion-/

Schmulson, M. (2015). Understanding bloating and distension. Retrieved October 30, 2015, from http://www.iffgd.org/site/manage-your-health/symptoms-causes/bloating-distension

Simpson, S., Ash, C., Pennisi, E., & Travis, J. (2005). The gut: inside out. *Science Magazine, 307*(5717), 1895. http://doi.org/DOI: 10.1126/science.307.5717.1895

Tresca, A. J. (2015). Normal bowel movements. Retrieved October 30, 2015, from http://ibdcrohns.about.com/od/dailylife/a/normalbm.htm

Vanderhoof, J. A., Pauley-Hunter, R. J., Lamont, J. T., & Grover, S. (2013). Treatment of small intestinal bacterial overgrowth. Retrieved October 30, 2015, from http://www.uptodate.com/contents/treatment-of-small-intestinal-bacterial-overgrowth?source=search_result&search=flatulence&selectedTitle=5~150

Vanderhoof, J. A., Pauley-Hunter, R. J., Lamont, J. T., & Grover, S. (2015). Chronic complications of the short bowel syndrome in adults http. Retrieved October 30, 2015, from http://www.uptodate.com/contents/chronic-complications-of-the-short-bowel-syndrome-in-adults?source=search_result&search=leaky+gut+syndrome&selectedTitle=4~109

Vanderhoof, J. A., Pauley-Hunter, R. J., Lamont, J. T., & Grover, S. (2015). Management of the short bowel syndrome in adults. Retrieved October 30, 2015, from http://www.uptodate.com/contents/management-of-the-short-bowel-syndrome-in-adults?source=search_result&search=leaky+gut+syndrome&selectedTitle=1~109

Vissera, J., Rozinga, J., Sapone, A., Lammers, K., & Fasano, A. (2009). Tight junctions, intestinal permeability, and autoimmunity celiac disease and type 1 diabetes paradigms. *Annals of the New York Academy of Sciences*, (1165), 195–205. http://doi.org/10.1111/j.1749-6632.2009.04037.x.

Wald, A., Talley, N. J., & Grover, S. (2015). Management of chronic constipation in adults. Retrieved October 30, 2015, from http://www.uptodate.com/contents/management-of-chronic-constipation-in-adults?source=search_result&search=constipation&selectedTitle=1~150

Wald, A., Talley, N. J., & Grover, S. (2014). Clinical manifestations and diagnosis of irritable bowel syndrome in adults. Retrieved October 30, 2015, from http://www.uptodate.com/contents/clinical-manifestations-and-diagnosis-of-irritable-bowel-syndrome-in-adults?source=search_result&search=flatulence&selectedTitle=9~150

Walter, S. A., Kjellström, L., Nyhlin, H., Talley, N. J., & Agréus, L. (2010). Assessment of normal bowel habits in the general adult population: the Popcol study. *Scandinavian Journal of Gastroenterology*, *45*(5), 556–66. http://doi.org/10.3109/00365520903551332

Medical Conditions

Alberta Cancer Prevention Legacy Fund. (2014). Backgrounder report: almost half of cancers in alberta are preventable.

Bacon, L., & Aphramor, L. (2011). Weight science: evaluating the evidence for a paradigm shift. *Nutrition Journal*, *10*(9). http://doi.org/10.1186/1475-2891-10-9

Becker, W., & Starrels, J. L. (2015). Prescription drug misuse: epidemiology, prevention, identification, and management. Retrieved October 25, 2015, from http://www.uptodate.com/contents/prescription-drug-misuse-epidemiology-prevention-identification-and-management?source=search_result&search=recreational+drugs+adult&selectedTitle=13~150

Bray, G. A. (2014). Obesity in adults: prevalence, screening, and evaluation. Retrieved October 25, 2015, from http://www.uptodate.com/contents/obesity-in-adults-prevalence-screening-and-evaluation?source=search_result&search=BMI&selectedTitle=2~150

Bray, G. A. (2015). Patient education: weight loss treatments (beyond the basics). Retrieved October 25, 2015, from http://www.uptodate.com/contents/weight-loss-treatments-beyond-the-basics?source=search_result&search=Weight+loss+treatments&selectedTitle=3~150

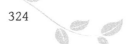

Bray, G. A. (2015). Obesity in adults: dietary therapy. Retrieved October 25, 2015, from http://www.uptodate.com/contents/obesity-in-adults-dietary-therapy?source=search_result&search=Obesity+in+adults%3A+Dietary+therapy&selectedTitle=1~150

Bystritsky, A. (2015). Complementary and alternative treatments for anxiety symptoms and disorders. Retrieved October 25, 2015, from http://www.uptodate.com/contents/complementary-and-alternative-treatments-for-anxiety-symptoms-and-disorders-physical-cognitive-and-spiritual-interventions?source=search_result&search=exercise&selectedTitle=9~150

Canada's Public Health Leader. (2008). *A tool for strengthening chronic disease prevention and management: through dialogue, planning and assessment.* Retrieved from http://www.cpha.ca/uploads/portals/cd/worksheets_e.pdf

Canadian Diabetes Association Clinical Practice Guidelines Expert Committee. (2013). Canadian diabetes association 2013 clinical practice guidelines for the prevention and management of diabetes in canada. *Canadian Journal of Diabetes*, 37(1), S1–S212. Retrieved from www.canadianjournalofdiabetes.com

Canadian Nurses Association. (2012). Effectiveness of registered nurses and nurse practitioners in supporting chronic disease self-management: a public health agency of canada funded project. Ottawa. Retrieved from http://www.cna-aiic.ca/

Conley, S., & Redeker, N. S. (2015). Cognitive behavioral therapy for insomnia in the context of cardiovascular conditions. *Current Sleep Medicine Reports, 1*, 157–165. http://doi.org/10.1007/s40675-015-0019-z

Dashti, H. M., Mathew, T. C., Khadada, M., Al-Mousawi, M., Talib, H., Asfar, S. K., … Al-Zaid, N. S. (2007). Beneficial effects of ketogenic diet in obese diabetic subjects. *Molecular and Cellular Biochemistry, 302*(1–2), 249–256. Retrieved from http://www.ncbi.nlm.nih.gov/pubmed/17447017

Fletcher, S. W., & Fletcher, R. H. (2015). Evidence-based approach to prevention. Retrieved October 25, 2015, from http://www.uptodate.com/contents/evidence-based-approach-to-prevention?source=search_result&search=health+screening&selectedTitle=6~150

Forhan, M., & Salas, X. R. (2013). Inequities in healthcare: a review of bias and discrimination in obesity treatment. *Canadian Journal of Diabetes, 37*, 205–209. http://doi.org/10.1016/j.jcjd.2013.03.362

Freedhoff, Y., & Sharma, A. M. (2010). *Best weight: a practical guide to office-based obesity management.* Canadian Obesity Network.

Freedhoff, Y., Sharma, A. M., Kirk, S. F. L., Vallis, M., Poirier, P., Ball, G. D. C., ... Christou, N. (2012). Realistic first steps for effectively managing obesity in canada. *Clinical Obesity, 2*, 78–82. http://doi.org/10.1111/j.1758-8111.2012.00044.x

Friedberg, M. W., & Landon, B. (2015). Measuring quality in hospitals in the united states. Retrieved January 26, 2016, from http://www.uptodate.com/contents/measuring-quality-in-hospitals-in-the-united-states?source=search_result&search=air+quality&selectedTitle=14~150

Frontline Health. (n.d.). Making the economic case for investing in public health and the sdh. Retrieved February 18, 2016, from http://www.cpha.ca/en/programs/social-determinants/frontlinehealth/economics.aspx

Hartigan, C., & Rainville, J. (2015). Exercise-based therapy for low back pain. Retrieved October 25, 2015, from http://www.uptodate.com/contents/exercise-based-therapy-for-low-back-pain?source=search_result&search=exercise&selectedTitle=17~150

Health Promotion and Disease Prevention in Canada. (2016). Chronic disease and injury indicator framework quick stats, 2016 edition (Vol. 36).

Hennekens, C. H. (2015). Overview of primary prevention of coronary heart disease and stroke. Retrieved October 25, 2015, from http://www.uptodate.com/contents/overview-of-primary-prevention-of-coronary-heart-disease-and-stroke?source=search_result&search=Overview+of+primary+prevention+of+coronary+heart+disease+and+stroke&selectedTitle=1~150

Huether, S. E., & McCance, K. L. (2008). *Understanding pathophysiology.* (V. L. Brashers & N. S. Rote, Eds.) (Fourth). St. Louis: Mosby Elsevier.

Institute of Medicine (US) Roundtable on Evidence-Based Medicine. (2010). *The healthcare imperative: lowering costs and improving outcomes: workshop series summary.* (P. L. Yong, R. S. Saunders, & L. A. Olsen, Eds.)*National Academy of Science.* Washington: National Academies Press. Retrieved from http://www.ncbi.nlm.nih.gov/books/NBK53914/

Jarvis, C. (2004). *Physical examination & health assessment* (Fourth). St. Louis: Saunders.

Kiel, D. P. (2015). Falls: prevention in community-dwelling older persons. Retrieved October 25, 2015, from http://www.uptodate.com/contents/falls-prevention-in-community-dwelling-older-persons?source=search_result&search=balance+training&selectedTitle=2~14

Kirk, S. F. L., & Penney, T. L. (2013). The role of health systems in obesity management and prevention: problems and paradigm shifts. *Current Obesity Reports, 2*(4), 315–319. http://doi.org/10.1007/s13679-013-0074-7

Lau, D. C. W., Douketis, J. D., Morrison, K. M., Hramiak, I. M., Sharma, A. M., & Ur, E. (2007). 2006 canadian clinical practice guidelines on the management and prevention of obesity in adults and children. *Canadian Medical Association Journal, 176*(8), 1–117. http://doi.org/10.1503/cmaj.061409

Marieb, E. N. (2004). *Human anatomy & physiology.* (M. A. Murray, W. Earl, & A. Wagner, Eds.) (Sixth). San Francisco: Pearson Benjamin Cummings.

McCulloch, D. K., & Robertson, R. P. (2015). Prevention of type 2 diabetes mellitus. Retrieved October 25, 2015, from http://www.uptodate.com/contents/prevention-of-type-2-diabetes-mellitus?source=search_result&search=prevention+of+type+2+diabetes&selectedTitle=1~150

Meigs, J. B. (2015). The metabolic syndrome (insulin resistance syndrome or syndrome X). Retrieved October 25, 2015, from http://www.uptodate.com/contents/the-metabolic-syndrome-insulin-resistance-syndrome-or-syndrome-x?source=search_result&search=waist+circumference&selectedTitle=4~111

O'Donnell, M. P. (2009). Definition of health promotion 2.0: embracing passion, enhancing motivation, recognizing dynamic balance, and creating opportunities. *American Journal of Health Promotion, Sept-Oct*(1). http://doi.org/10.4278/ajhp.24.1.iv

Park, L. (2015). Preventive care in adults: recommendations. Retrieved October 25, 2015, from http://www.uptodate.com/contents/preventive-care-in-adults-recommendations?source=search_result&search=health+screening&selectedTitle=1~150

Reel, J. J., Stuart, A. R., & Reel, J. (2012). Is the "health at every size" approach useful for addressing obesity? *Community Medicine & Health Education Reel and Stuart J Community Med Health Educ J Community Med Health Educ, 2*(4), 1–2. http://doi.org/10.4172/2161-0711.1000e105

Rosenquist, E. W. K. (2015). Overview of the treatment of chronic pain. Retrieved October 25, 2015, from http://www.uptodate.com/contents/overview-of-the-treatment-of-chronic-pain?source=search_result&search=pain&selectedTitle=1~150

Sainsbury, A., & Hay, P. (2014). Correction: call for an urgent rethink of the "health at every size" concept. *Journal of Eating Disorders, 2*(13), 1–2. http://doi.org/10.1186/2050-2974-2-13

Seal, N. (2011). Introduction to genetics and childhood obesity: relevance to nursing practice. *Biological Research for Nursing, 13*(1), 61–9. http://doi.org/10.1177/1099800410381424

Sharma, A. M. (2010). M, m, m & m: a mnemonic for assessing obesity. *Obesity Reviews, 11*, 808–9. http://doi.org/10.1111/j.1467-789X.2010.00766.x

Sheehan, N. C., & Yin, L. (2006). Childhood obesity: nursing policy implications. *Journal of Pediatric Nursing, 21*(4), 308–10. http://doi.org/10.1016/j.pedn.2006.04.001

Tylka, T. L., Annunziato, R. A., Burgard, D., Daníelsdóttir, S., Shuman, E., Davis, C., & Calogero, R. (2014). The weight-inclusive versus weight-normative approach to health: evaluating the evidence for prioritizing well-being over weight loss. *Journal of Obesity, 2014*, 1–18. http://doi.org/10.1155/2014/983495

Whiting, C., Brown, S., Alvi, R., & Tonita, J. (2010). A call to action for a cancer prevention plan for saskatchewan: a proposal for discussion - summary. Retrieved from www.saskcancer.ca

Wilson, J. L. (2001). *Adrenal fatigue: the 21st century stress syndrome* (First). Petaluma: Smart Publications.

Wolin, K. Y., & Colditz, G. A. (2014). Cancer prevention. Retrieved June 21, 2015, from http://www.uptodate.com/contents/cancer-prevention?source=search_result&search=cancer+prevention&selectedTitle=1~150

Woolhandler, S., Campbell, T., & Himmelstein, D. A. U. (2003). Costs of health care administration in the united states and canada. *New England Journal of Medicine, 349*, 768–75.

Yates, T., Haffner, S. M., Schulte, P. J., Thomas, L., Huffman, K. M., Bales, C. W., ... Kraus, W. E. (2013). Association between change in daily ambulatory activity and cardiovascular events in people with impaired glucose tolerance (NAVIGATOR trial): a cohort analysis. *The Lancet, 383*, 1059–1066. http://doi.org/http://dx.doi.org/10.1016/S0140-6736(13)62061-9

Preventing chronic disease strategic plan 2013-2016. (2013).

Chronic disease related to aging: brief to the house of commons standing committee on health. (2011). Ottawa. Retrieved from https://cna-aiic.ca/~/media/cna/page-content/pdf-en/hesa_brief_on_chronic_disease_and_aging_e.pdf?la=en

Lifestyle Factors

Agarwal, K. (2015). Failure to thrive in elderly adults: management. Retrieved January 26, 2016, from http://www.uptodate.com/contents/failure-to-thrive-in-elderly-adults-management?source=search_result&search=marijuana&selectedTitle=21~150

Agronin, M. (2014). Sexual dysfunction in older adults. Retrieved January 26, 2016, from http://www.uptodate.com/contents/sexual-dysfunction-in-older-adults?source=search_result&search=safe+sex+practices&selectedTitle=8~150

Ahasic, A., & Redlich, C. A. (2014). Building related air quality. Retrieved January 26, 2016, from http://www.uptodate.com/contents/building-related-illness-and-building-related-symptoms?source=search_result&search=fresh+air&selectedTitle=1~150

Baron, E. D. (2015). Selection of sunscreen and sun protective measures. Retrieved January 26, 2016, from http://www.uptodate.com/contents/selection-of-sunscreen-and-sun-protective-measures?source=search_result&search=sun+exposure&selectedTitle=3~150

Becker, W., & Starrels, J. L. (2015). Prescription drug misuse: epidemiology, prevention, identification, and management. Retrieved January 26, 2016, from http://www.uptodate.com/contents/prescription-drug-misuse-epidemiology-prevention-identification-and-management?source=search_result&search=recreational+drugs+adult&selectedTitle=13~150

Ben-Sefer, E. (2009). The childhood obesity pandemic: promoting knowledge for undergraduate nursing students. *Nurse Education in Practice*, *9*(3), 159–65. http://doi.org/10.1016/j.nepr.2008.07.006

Betancourt, J. R., Green, A. R., & Carrillo, J. E. (2014). Cross cultural care and communication. Retrieved January 26, 2016, from http://www.uptodate.com/contents/cross-cultural-care-and-communication?source=search_result&search=family+dynamics&selectedTitle=4~150

Borradaile, K. E., Sherman, S., Vander Veur, S. S., McCoy, T., Sandoval, B., Nachmani, J., ... Foster, G. D. (2009). Snacking in children: the role of urban corner stores. *Pediatrics*, *124*(5), 1293–8. http://doi.org/10.1542/peds.2009-0964

Casamassimo, P. S. (2015). Oral and systemic health. Retrieved January 26, 2016, from http://www.uptodate.com/contents/oral-and-systemic-health?source=search_result&search=dental+health&selectedTitle=2~150

Cowan, E., & Su, M. (2015). Ethanol intoxication in adults. Retrieved January 26, 2016, from http://www.uptodate.com/contents/ethanol-intoxication-in-adults?source=search_result&search=alchohol&selectedTitle=3~150

Curiel-Lewandrowski, C. (2015). Risk factors for the development of melanoma. Retrieved January 26, 2016, from http://www.uptodate.com/contents/risk-factors-for-the-development-of-melanoma?source=search_result&search=sun+exposure&selectedTitle=6~150up

Dammann, K. W., & Smith, C. (2010). Race, homelessness, and other environmental factors associated with the food-purchasing behavior of low-income women. *Journal of the American Dietetic Association, 110*(9), 1351–6. http://doi.org/10.1016/j.jada.2010.06.007

Frank, D. A., Neault, N. B., Skalicky, A., Cook, J. T., Wilson, J. D., Levenson, S., ... Berkowitz, C. (2006). Heat or eat: the low income home energy assistance program and nutritional and health risks among children less than 3 years of age. *Pediatrics, 118*(5), e1293-302. http://doi.org/10.1542/peds.2005-2943

French, S. A., Wall, M., & Mitchell, N. R. (2010). Household income differences in food sources and food items purchased. *The International Journal of Behavioral Nutrition and Physical Activity, 7*(1), 77. http://doi.org/10.1186/1479-5868-7-77

Fryar, C. D., Gu, Q., & Ogden, C. L. (2012). Anthropometric reference data for children and adults: united states 2007-2010. Vital Health Stat (Vol. 11).

Gay, C. L., & Cohen, M. S. (2015). Prevention of sexually transmitted infections. Retrieved January 26, 2016, from http://www.uptodate.com/contents/prevention-of-sexually-transmitted-infections?source=search_result&search=safe+sex+practices&selectedTitle=1~150

Goldman, R. H. (2015). Information and educational resources for occupational and environmental health issues in the United States. Retrieved January 26, 2016, from http://www.uptodate.com/contents/information-and-educational-resources-for-occupational-and-environmental-health-issues-in-the-united-states?source=search_result&search=environmental+toxins&selectedTitle=1~36

Kirkpatrick, S., & Tarasuk, V. (2003). The relationship between low income and household food expenditure patterns in Canada. *Public Health Nutrition, 6*(6), 589–597. http://doi.org/10.1079/PHN2003517

Lorenzini, A. (2014). How much should we weigh for a long and healthy life span? The need to reconcile caloric restriction versus longevity with body mass index versus mortality data. *Frontiers in Endocrinology*, 5(121), 1–8. http://doi.org/10.3389/fendo.2014.00121

Mannino, D. M. (2015). Cigarette smoking and other risk factors for lung cancer. Retrieved January 26, 2016, from http://www.uptodate.com/contents/cigarette-smoking-and-other-risk-factors-for-lung-cancer?source=search_result&search=smoking&selectedTitle=3~150

Mukamal, K. J. (2015). Overview of the risks and benefits of alcohol consumption. Retrieved January 26, 2016, from http://www.uptodate.com/contents/overview-of-the-risks-and-benefits-of-alcohol-consumption?source=search_result&search=alcohol&selectedTitle=2~150

Nelson, M. C., & Story, M. (2009). Food environments in university dorms: 20,000 calories per dorm room and counting. *American Journal of Preventive Medicine*, 36(6), 523–6. http://doi.org/10.1016/j.amepre.2009.01.030

Peterman, A. H., Rothrock, N., & Cella, D. (2015). Evaluation of health related quality of life (HRQL) in patients with a serious life-threatening illness. Retrieved January 26, 2016, from http://www.uptodate.com/contents/evaluation-of-health-related-quality-of-life-hrql-in-patients-with-a-serious-life-threatening-illness?source=search_result&search=air+quality&selectedTitle=3~150

Raby, B. A. (2015). Personalized medicine. Retrieved January 26, 2016, from http://www.uptodate.com/contents/personalized-medicine?source=search_result&search=epigenetics&selectedTitle=1~16

Ricciuto, L., Tarasuk, V., & Yatchew, A. (2006). Socio-demographic influences on food purchasing among canadian households. *European Journal of Clinical Nutrition*, 60(6), 778–90. http://doi.org/10.1038/sj.ejcn.1602382

Rigotti, N. A. (2015). Benefits and risks of smoking cessation. Retrieved October 25, 2015, from http://www.uptodate.com/contents/benefits-and-risks-of-smoking-cessation?source=search_result&search=smoking&selectedTitle=4~150

Rosenquist, E. W. K. (2015). Overview of the treatment of chronic pain. Retrieved January 26, 2016, from http://www.uptodate.com/contents/overview-of-the-treatment-of-chronic-pain?source=search_result&search=marijuana&selectedTitle=13~150

Saitz, R. (2015). Screening for unhealthy use of alcohol and other drugs in primary care. Retrieved January 26, 2016, from http://www.uptodate.com/contents/screening-for-unhealthy-use-of-alcohol-and-other-drugs-in-primary-care?source=search_result&search=recreational+drugs+adult&selectedTitle=12~150

Samet, J. M., & Sockrider, M. (2015). Control of secondhand smoke exposure. Retrieved January 26, 2016, from http://www.uptodate.com/contents/control-of-secondhand-smoke-exposure?source=search_result&search=air+quality&selectedTitle=18~150

Sisk, C., Sharkey, J. R., McIntosh, W. A., & Anding, J. (2010). Using multiple household food inventories to measure food availability in the home over 30 days: a pilot study. *Nutrition Journal, 9*, 19. http://doi.org/10.1186/1475-2891-9-19

Sutherland, L. A., Beavers, D. P., Kupper, L. L., Bernhardt, A. M., Heatherton, T., & Dalton, M. A. (2008). Like parent, like child: child food and beverage choices during role playing. *Archives of Pediatrics & Adolescent Medicine, 162*(11), 1063–9. http://doi.org/10.1001/archpedi.162.11.1063

Sutin, A. R., Ferrucci, L., Zonderman, A. B., & Terracciano, A. (2011). Personality and obesity across the adult lifespan. *Journal of Personality and Social Psychology, 101*(3), 579–592. http://doi.org/10.1037/a0024286

Wiecha, J. L., Finkelstein, D., Troped, P. J., Fragala, M., & Peterson, K. E. (2006). School vending machine use and fast-food restaurant use are associated with sugar-sweetened beverage intake in youth. *Journal of the American Dietetic Association, 106*(10), 1624–30. http://doi.org/10.1016/j.jada.2006.07.007

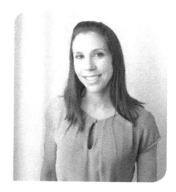

About the Author

*S*hawna Curry, RN, BN, B.KIN, CTI Co-Active Coach, has over fifteen years of experience in the world of health as a Registered Nurse, Professional Coach, Author, Public Speaker, Personal Trainer, Endurance Training Coach, and Fitness Instructor. Thanks to her varied experience, Shawna is able to provide clients with an experience that is intimate, informative, and inspiring.

Shawna brings personal experience from years of doing triathlons and marathons while dealing with food sensitivities, inflammation, and multiple sports injuries. She has learned how to overcome feelings of being broken and uses this experience to teach others how to take charge of their own health in order to achieve optimal health.

Shawna has presented at the CARNA100 Conference in conjunction with Neil Pasricha, author of *The Happiness Equation*, and Paul Brandt, Juno-winning Canadian country artist. She has also done numerous presentations for the Running Room, Lupus Society of Alberta, Alberta Health Services Women's Health Resources, Canadian Firefighters Hockey Club, Momentum Health Calgary, and the Tech Shop. Her writing has been published in *Forbes Science, Inc.,* and *Impact* magazines.

Shawna is on a mission to inspire others to be proactive and preventive with their health. You can find out more about Shawna and her current work on her website at www.yourlifestylestrategy.com.

CPSIA information can be obtained
at www.ICGtesting.com
Printed in the USA
LVHW012031190720
661002LV00014B/381